616.89 EXAM   LAN

New MRCPsych Paper I Mock MCQ Papers

To all my teachers.

New MRCPsych Paper I Mock MCQ Papers

VELLINGIRI BADRAKALIMUTHU

MBBS, MRCPsych
Speciality Registrar in Old Age Psychiatry
PBL Tutor for ST1 & ST2 Psychiatry Trainees
Norfolk and Waveney Mental Health Foundation NHS Trust
Julian Hospital, Norwich

Foreword by

HUGO de WAAL

MD, FRCPsych
Head of School, Postgraduate School of Psychiatry
East of England Deanery
College Tutor, Norfolk & Waveney Psychiatric Training Scheme
Fellow, Higher Education Academy

Radcliffe Publishing
Oxford • New York

Radcliffe Publishing Ltd
18 Marcham Road
Abingdon
Oxon OX14 1AA
United Kingdom

www.radcliffe-oxford.com
Electronic catalogue and worldwide online ordering facility.

British Library Cataloguing in Publication Data

A catalogue record for this book is available from the British Library.

ISBN-13: 978 184619 313 2

Typeset by Pindar NZ, Auckland, New Zealand
Printed and bound by TJI Digital, Padstow, Cornwall, UK

Contents

Foreword

As college tutor I have been trying for some years to get the message through to trainees that, although passing the College exams is an essential part of their path towards achieving the status of 'expert', they should never forget that there is more to becoming an expert than managing to pass exams. We all know (and perhaps envy) colleagues who passed on their first attempt with apparently less effort than we had to put in ourselves, whereas others, who seem perfectly trustworthy clinicians, struggle and fail regardless of how much time and effort they put into their preparation.

So what is the point of exams and, by extension, of this book?

Perhaps it would help to concentrate the mind, by reminding ourselves of the varied fortunes of a now largely forgotten English cleric, Charles Caleb Colton (1780–1832). Having been appointed to the perpetual curacy of Tiverton's Prior's Quarter in Devon at the age of 21, he fluctuated between displaying a hard-working brilliance at some times with a drifting neglect of his church duties at others, the latter leading to limiting the concept of 'in perpetuity' in his case to a mere 10 years! As with many brilliant minds he suffered from too wide a range of hobbies: apparently he had to flee from England after defaulting on debts accrued as a not-so-successful wine merchant: a less obvious activity for a churchman than might seem to emanate from the Eucharist. If anyone had a grasp on how to deal with failing, it must have been he:

> *'Examinations are formidable even to the best prepared, for the greatest fool may ask more than the wisest man can answer.'*

Colton's wisdom provides a method of dealing with the feeling of irritation that often descends on candidates preparing for the College exams: just think about the foolishness of those who set the exams!

Anyone sufficiently brilliant to reach the point of sitting the exams cannot help but smile benignly and get on with the task of proving to the fools that you are better than they are.

Nevertheless, the author of this book still took into account the distant possibility that the exam designers *do* know what they are doing: hence, all questions and answers have been tested on our own trainees and validated in the workplace. Feedback suggested that the book provided a thorough preparation for the exams and this was borne out by the high pass rates achieved by that particular sample of candidates. Needless to say, the answers have been carefully cross-referenced.

Criticism of examinations probably originated at the time when the first-ever candidate failed the first-ever exam: 'you are never tested on the issues that really matter', 'once you have passed you will never again use the vast bulk of the knowledge acquired', etc. These lead us back to considering the nature of an 'expert': an expert knows far more than is needed in the routine practice of the field of expertise. The rub lies in the term 'routine'. Virtually anyone can be trained to deal with routine matters, but it is the expert who can be relied upon when the problem transcends the ordinary. For the expert therefore, there is no such thing as irrelevant knowledge and it is with that insight in mind that the information in this volume should be absorbed. Or to quote Bertrand Russell:

'There is much pleasure to be gained from useless knowledge.'

So, enjoy!!

Hugo de Waal MD, FRCPsych
Head of School, Postgraduate School of Psychiatry,
East of England Deanery
College Tutor, Norfolk & Waveney
Psychiatric Training Scheme
Fellow, Higher Education Academy
September 2008

Preface

The Royal College of Psychiatrists has made significant changes to the examination format and has adopted MCQ papers as a test of theoretical knowledge. MCQs are in the format of 'single best answer from five' style. In a 200-question paper, about two-thirds comprise MCQs and one-third EMIs (Extended Matching Items).

This book of mock tests is an attempt to simulate exam conditions using questions derived from factual data contained in books recommended for the MRCPsych Paper 1.

The MRCPsych Paper 1 will contain questions on the following topics:

- General adult
- History and mental state examination
- Cognitive assessment
- Neurological examination
- Assessment
- Aetiology
- Diagnosis
- Classification
- Basic psychopharmacology
- Basic psychological processes
- Human psychological development
- Social psychology
- Description and measurement
- Basic psychological treatments
- Prevention of psychiatric disorder
- Descriptive psychopathology

- Dynamic psychopathology
- History of psychiatry
- Basic ethics and philosophy of psychiatry
- Stigma and culture

The author of this book has looked closely at these topics and produced questions that have been tested on the ST1 Psychiatry trainees involved with the Norfolk & Waveney Mental Health Foundation NHS Trust. The questions have been complimented for offering factual knowledge without losing focus on the exam. Every effort has been made to ensure accuracy of the information provided. However, the trainees are advised to read through references quoted to ensure a comprehensive understanding of the question themes.

The book does not provide explanatory answers because the questions are based on books quoted in reference elsewhere and should be used as sign posts for trainees to read the relevant references and gain further knowledge.

Success in examinations needs dedicated preparation, and from my experience there is no substitute for hard work.

Vellingiri Badrakalimuthu
September 2008

About the author

Having completed MBBS at Coimbatore Medical College, India in 2002, Vellingiri trained in psychiatry at the Institute of Mental Health, Chennai, India. His first appointment in UK was at the Maudsley Hospital following which he was a senior house officer on Solent rotation. He became a Member of the Royal College of Psychiatrists in 2007. He is currently pursuing a masters degree in neuroscience at the Institute of Psychiatry, King's College, London.

He has many research publications to his credit and was commissioned by the *British Medical Journal* to review evidence for treatments in acute schizophrenia. He also represented the Royal College of Psychiatrists at the BMJ Career Fair in 2006. He is currently a speciality registrar in old age psychiatry in Norwich and also serves as the Problem-Based Learning Tutor for first and second year trainees in psychiatry. He also organises psychopharmacology training days for psychiatry trainees in Eastern Deanery.

Paper 1

1. A 6-month-old infant fails to retrieve a rattle covered by a cloth. According to Piaget the child is at the:
   a. Preoperational stage
   b. Concrete operational stage
   c. Sensorimotor stage
   d. Formal operational stage
   e. Properational stage

2. Two cloths labelled A and B are placed side by side on a table and a rattle is put under cloth A on three successive trials. On the fourth trial it is placed under cloth B but the watching infant perseveres in searching under cloth A. This is an example of:
   a. Missing points of view
   b. Perception subordinate to action
   c. Non-logical thought
   d. Hypothesising
   e. Distinguishing self and not-self

3. With regard to the deceptive box test which of the following is true?
   a. A 3-year-old child will be able to predict another child's behaviour
   b. A similar imaginative bicycle test was devised by Wellman and Estes
   c. Failure is indicative of egocentrism
   d. It can be successfully performed by an autistic child
   e. It is not used to test theory of mind

4. In the Little Albert test, a metal bar is struck behind a child's ear. Which of the following is a correct statement?
   a. The noise from the metal bar is a conditioned stimulus
   b. The noise leads to an unconditioned response
   c. The amount of overt behaviour is a measure of the association between rat and fear
   d. The test is an example of instrumental conditioning
   e. None of the above

5. The theory of working memory was developed by:
   a. Tulving
   b. Anderson
   c. Baddeley
   d. Craik and Lockhart
   e. Milner

6. The most important factor that helps memory in its application to Problem-Based Learning (PBL) is:
   a. Organisation
   b. Integration
   c. Elaboration
   d. Schemata
   e. Super memory

7. In the Ames room experiment, people are observed to shrink and grow because of:
   a. Size constancy
   b. Three-dimensional constancy
   c. Shape constancy
   d. Vertical drop
   e. Horizontal drop

8. An FY2 trainee in Psychiatry with no interest in Psychiatry continues the job because of the pay. This is known as:
   a. Fixed interval reinforcement

b. Fixed ratio reinforcement

c. Variable interval reinforcement

d. Variable ratio reinforcement

e. Altruism

9. The loss of sense of personal identity and autobiographical memory is:
   a. Organic amnesia
   b. Not the fugue state
   c. An example of infantile amnesia
   d. Anterograde amnesia
   e. Unrelated to any of the above

10. A child can tell that a tall glass and a wide-mouthed narrow glass of equal volume hold the same amount of water. According to Piaget, the child is at the:
    a. Sensorimotor stage
    b. Preoperational stage
    c. Concrete operational stage
    d. Formal operation stage
    e. Properational stage

11. With regard to the psychometric approach which of the following is not a disadvantage?
    a. It is theoretical
    b. It lacks a driving theory of cognition
    c. It relies on statistical measures hindering establishing relationship between Central Nervous System (CNS) structure and function
    d. Some redundant information is produced
    e. It allows the misconception that it is easy to access brain function

12. Performance sub-sets of WAIS-R include all but
    a. Picture completion
    b. Digit span
    c. Picture arrangement
    d. Digit symbol
    e. Block design

13. The WMS-R assesses all but
    a. Information and orientation
    b. Mental control
    c. Comprehension
    d. Paired associate learning
    e. Visual paired associates

14. Which one of these statements is correct with regard to dissatisfaction and social exchange?
    a. Loyalty is a response to dissatisfaction
    b. Investment and commitment are significant factors when taken together with satisfaction and alternatives
    c. The difference between unhappy couples is greater for verbal behaviour
    d. Four dysfunctional beliefs include that mind reading is expected
    e. One dysfunctional belief is that the sexes are the same

15. Which one of these statements is correct with regard to personality assessment?
    a. The disadvantage of Eysenck's model is that it is restricted to Western civilisation
    b. Personality dimension psychosis measures the actual psychological disorder
    c. Eysenck's model is hierarchical
    d. Night skin conductance is higher in introverts than in extroverts
    e. Personality trait E maps on to histrionic, narcissistic and passive-aggressive personality disorders

16. Which one of these statements is correct with regard to gender differences?
    a. The majority of adults on treatment for a psychological disorder are men
    b. Gender has sociological connotations
    c. Boys are more aggressive than girls on the physical but not the verbal dimension
    d. Girls are more suggestible than boys
    e. Freud suggested that internalisation of gender occurs at a very early age

17. Which of the following statements is correct with regard to personality and gender?
    a. There is a lack of relationship between extreme helplessness and dependency of the agoraphobic, and the social expectations for women
    b. Learned helplessness is an explanation for higher rates of depression in men
    c. In depressive personality, passivity, dependence and lack of self-confidence is the intensification of normal female characteristics
    d. There is no gender-based difference in the ways distress is expressed
    e. None of the above is true

18. Which one of these statements about studies on adversity is correct?
    a. Goal-frustration is associated with depression
    b. There is an additive effect of adverse events leading up to depression
    c. In depression compared to schizophrenia, the number of adverse events increases in the three weeks prior to relapse
    d. 20% of women experiencing adverse events go on to develop a depressive disorder
    e. Brown and Harris found that having four or more young children predisposed people to depression

19. Jamie, travelling on a train for the first time, notices that the trees outside appear to be travelling in the opposite direction to the moving train. What is this phenomenon known as?
    a. Figure-ground differentiation
    b. Motion parallax
    c. Location constancy
    d. Divergence
    e. Convergence

20. A psychologist takes Mr Taylor, who has had a fear of heights, to the top of Spinnaker Tower in Portsmouth. What is this therapy called?
    a. Implosion
    b. Flooding
    c. Relaxation training
    d. Desensitisation
    e. Imaginable flooding

21. Which one of the following is a short, self-reporting personality test that has dimensional scales and has been validated in non-clinical populations?
    a. EPQ
    b. 16 PF Q
    c. MMPI-2
    d. PAI
    e. IPDE

22. When Manchester United and Arsenal compete for the Premiership title, fans become prejudiced against each other. What is the term for this?
    a. Frustration-aggression hypothesis
    b. Social identity theory
    c. Realistic conflict
    d. Fraternalistic deprivation
    e. Racism

23. Thirty-month-old Amy points at a Kit-Kat bar at a newsagent and shouts, 'Chocolate want,' using two words together for first time. This development is:
   a. Later than one would expect for the child's age
   b. Earlier than one would expect for the child's age
   c. At the lower limit of the range of normal development
   d. At the upper limit of the range of normal development
   e. None of the above

24. A young African-Caribbean male admitted to the PICU, sat facing away from the clinical team when invited to a ward round. This is known as:
   a. Obstruction
   b. Somatic passivity
   c. Resistance
   d. Stereotypy
   e. Negativism

25. A 69-year-old man with depression believes that he is in danger of imminent arrest for murder despite never having committed a crime. This condition is known as:
   a. Delusion of guilt
   b. Delusion of reference
   c. Depersonalisation
   d. Nihilistic delusion
   e. Anhedonia

26. A 43-year-old woman, who miraculously survived a serious accident on the M1 believed, at the time of the accident, that the world had ceased to exist. This is known as:
   a. Derealisation
   b. Depersonalisation
   c. Nihilistic delusion
   d. Suicidal thought
   e. None of the above

27. Mr Allen, a scriptwriter for Universal Studios, had a long history of bipolar affective disorder. He had been increasingly agitated on the run-up to this year's Oscars and on the day of the ceremony he said that the red carpet appeared to be more vivid and bright, and that the cheers from the crowd were louder than thousands of pneumatic drills. This condition is known as:
    a. Dysmegalopsia
    b. Macropsia
    c. Hyperaesthesia
    d. Illusion
    e. Oneiroid state

28. James was worried that he had to shout 'Jordan' whenever he saw an attractive woman, despite his best efforts to keep calm. This shows:
    a. Somatic passivity
    b. A made act
    c. A compulsive image
    d. An obsessional impulse
    e. A first rank symptom of schizophrenia

29. The ability to answer MCQs primarily involves:
    a. Registration
    b. Retention
    c. Recognition
    d. Rehearsal
    e. None of the above

30. Which of the following is a false statement regarding primary memory?
    a. It is also known as short-term memory
    b. It lasts for 30 seconds when items are rehearsed
    c. Only about six to eight items can be stored
    d. Digit span is a test of this function
    e. It is also known as working memory

31. In the palimpsest, the following type of memory loss is seen:
    a. Retrograde amnesia
    b. Anterograde amnesia due to failure of recall
    c. Anterograde amnesia due to failure of registration
    d. Both retrograde and anterograde amnesia
    e. Apperception

32. Which among the following is not a part of Mini-Mental State Examination?
    a. Serial sevens test
    b. Digit span test
    c. 3-item recall test
    d. 3-stage command test
    e. 2-item naming test

33. Damage to the hippocampal region is a feature of all, except:
    a. Post-herpetic encephalitis
    b. Bilateral temporal lobe operations
    c. Impairment of retrieval
    d. Korsakoff's syndrome
    e. Preserved insight

34. All the following are sensory distortions, except:
    a. Hyperaesthesia
    b. Hypoacusis
    c. Dysmegalopsia
    d. Macropsia
    e. Pseudo hallucination

35. All the following are types of Wernicke's aphasia, except:
    a. Transcortical aphasia
    b. Pure word deafness
    c. Agnostic alexia
    d. Receptive aphasia
    e. Visual asymbolia

36. Characteristics of preconscious thinking include all, except:
   a. Outside awareness
   b. Secondary process thinking
   c. Image orientation
   d. Accessible through focussed attention
   e. The reality principle

37. Characteristics of 'unconscious' include all, except:
   a. Linear
   b. Word oriented
   c. Denotative
   d. Timelessness
   e. Secondary process thinking

38. 'Latent dream' includes all, except:
   a. Symbolism
   b. Day residue
   c. Unconscious wishes
   d. Dream work
   e. Nocturnal stimuli

39. 'I thought that my life was outside my feet and made my feet vibrate.' This is known as:
   a. Kinaesthetic hallucination
   b. Somatic passivity
   c. Haptic hallucination
   d. Delusion of control
   e. Made feeling

40. Formication is a type of:
   a. Superficial hallucination
   b. Haptic hallucination
   c. Kinaesthetic hallucination

d. Visceral hallucination

e. Delusional infestation

41. Which one these statements about pseudo hallucination is not true?

    a. It is indefinite, incomplete only individual details

    b. It is retained

    c. It cannot be dismissed

    d. It is relevant to emotions

    e. It is subjective

42. Capgras' syndrome is:

    a. A perceptual abnormality

    b. A form of autoscopy

    c. A form of negative autoscopy

    d. Also called the phantom mirror image

    e. A delusional misidentification

43. A schizophrenic patient heard hallucinatory voices only when water flowed from tap. This is:

    a. Delusional perception

    b. Delusional misinterpretation

    c. Functional hallucination

    d. Reflex hallucination

    e. Hygric hallucination

44. The following is innate:

    a. Colour constancy

    b. Visual constancy

    c. Size constancy

    d. Orientation constancy

    e. Figure-ground constancy

45. Attention can be measured by:

    a. The Serial Seven test

    b. Reciting months of a year in the reverse order

    c. Using the Stroop test

    d. Spelling WORLD in reverse

    e. All of the above

46. The type of memory that is part of long-term memory includes:

    a. Episodic memory

    b. Primary memory

    c. Sensory memory

    d. Motor memory

    e. Working memory

47. Functions of the prefrontal cortex include all, except:

    a. Problem solving

    b. Perceptual judgement

    c. Verbal regulation

    d. Personality

    e. Memory

48. Frontal lobe damage:

    a. Causes contralateral spastic paresis

    b. Causes ipsilateral spastic paresis

    c. Does not cause spastic paresis

    d. Causes contralateral hypotonia

    e. Causes ipsilateral hypotonia

49. The presence of an observer changes the outcome of an experiment. This is due to:

    a. Halo effect

    b. Hawthorne effect

    c. Response set

d. Extreme responding

e. Reliability error

50. A 39-year-old man can be tested for IQ using:
   a. WISC-R
   b. WMS-R
   c. WPPSI
   d. WAIS-R
   e. Stanford-Binet test

51. The projective test of personality is:
   a. 16-PF
   b. MMPI
   c. California Psychological Inventory
   d. IPDE
   e. TAT

52. The use of private language is known as:
   a. Cryptographia
   b. Neologism
   c. Logoclonia
   d. Echolalia
   e. Paragrammatism

53. Mr Grant presents with normal spontaneous speech, comprehension and repetition, but has impaired naming, reading and writing ability. This is known as:
   a. Pure word blindness
   b. Pure word dumbness
   c. Transcortical motor dysphasia
   d. Alexia with agraphia
   e. Transcortical sensory dysphasia

54. Which of these is a form of agnosia?

    a. Subcortical visual aphasia

    b. Isolated speech area dysphasia

    c. Transcortical sensory dysphasia

    d. Transcortical motor dysphasia

    e. Conduction dysphasia

55. The following associations are true, except:

    a. Bleuler – loosening of associations

    b. Goldstein – asyndesis

    c. Schneider – drivelling

    d. Kraepelin – acataphasia

    e. Mortimer – formal thought disorder is a disorder of semantic memory

56. Choose the true definition:

    a. Alogia – intrusion of irrelevant or bizarre thought

    b. Paraphasia – positive thought disorder

    c. Verbal paraphasia – loss of appropriate word but sentences are meaningful

    d. Telegramese – loss of adverbs

    e. Paralogia – loss of grammatism

57. The following are somatic and autonomic symptoms of anxiety, except:

    a. Palpitations

    b. Insomnia

    c. Dizziness

    d. Difficulty in breathing

    e. Abdominal churning

58. Anxiety may be a direct expression of morbid process in all, except:

    a. Hypoglycaemia

    b. Hyperparathyroidism

c. Hyperthyroidism

d. Phaeochromocytoma

e. Carcinoid syndrome

59. A woman who saw corpses in coffins had to imagine the same people standing. This is known as:

a. Obsessional image

b. Compulsive image

c. Disaster image

d. Disruptive image

e. Rumination

60. Irritability and aggression is commonly seen in:

a. Hypothyroidism

b. Hypoxia

c. Hyperglycaemia

d. Hyperparathyroidism

e. All of the above

61. According to the psychiatric classification of arson, fire setting for avoiding the detection of crime is:

a. Revenge fire setting

b. Fire setting for pleasure and excitement

c. Political arson

d. Profitable arson

e. Accidental fire setting

62. The effects of drugs on sensorimotor performance can be studied by:

a. CFF

b. Stabilometer

c. Paper and pencil tests

d. Gibson spiral maze test

e. Finger tapping test

63. A condition that shows low placebo response is:

   a. Conversion state

   b. Dysthymia

   c. Manic episode

   d. Drug-induced psychosis

   e. Anxiety disorder

64. Depressive symptoms that favour a response to antidepressant drugs include all, except:

   a. Hopelessness

   b. Guilt

   c. Motor agitation

   d. Early insomnia

   e. Anhedonia

65. Which of the following is true with regard to treating side-effects from psychotropics?

   a. Polyuria associated with lithium can be treated with carbamazepine

   b. Impaired ejaculation from SSRIs can be treated with cyproheptadine

   c. Leucopenia associated with clozapine can be treated with carbamazepine

   d. Excessive sweating from tricyclics can be treated with beta-blockers

   e. Impaired erection from tricyclics can be treated with neostigmine

66. During an inpatient admission, a 37-year-old man has his dose of antipsychotic drug increased. Following this, he develops fever, sweating, agitation and rigidity. One among the following will influence your management plan:

   a. Renal function tests will confirm your diagnosis

   b. Most common cause is delirium from dehydration due to negative symptoms

   c. Mortality rate is 20–30%

d. In the future, do not start him on antipsychotics

e. Liver function tests will confirm the diagnosis

67. Mr Anderson has a history of alcohol dependence. He suffers from skin conditions especially when his dependence becomes worse. He has recently been diagnosed with depression by a nurse practitioner and has been started on a particular antidepressant. Since then, his GP has phoned up to say that the patient has a flared-up skin rash. What could be the antidepressant?

a. Citalopram

b. Sertraline

c. Paroxetine

d. Fluoxetine

e. Fluvoxamine

68. A 36-year-old-barrister had recently completed a detox for alcohol dependence. She was started on relapse prevention measures including biological treatments. Her husband was so pleased with her success that he bought her a new perfume. On using this she immediately developed nausea and flushing, and upon attempting to stand from her sitting position she promptly fell down. Which one of the following medications is likely to be the cause?

a. Acamprosate

b. Moclobemide

c. Disulfiram

d. Naltrexone

e. Chlordiazepoxide

69. A 28-year-old homeless man underwent an emergency detox after he was found by the roadside suffering from alcohol withdrawal. He had developed delirium tremens during this episode. During detox he developed painful fingers, especially when he tried to warm them. On examination, he had very pale fingers. Which of these medications is likely to be implicated?

   a. Chlordiazepoxide

   b. Clomethiazole

   c. Diazepam

   d. Clonidine

   e. Acamprosate

70. A 22-year-old lady, who was started on olanzapine following a presentation with paranoia and auditory hallucinations, complains of drowsiness and weight gain. This is due to blocking of:

   a. Alpha-1 and histamine-2 receptors

   b. Alpha-1 and histamine-1 receptors

   c. Serotonergic and dopamine receptors

   d. Alpha-2 and histamine-2 receptors

   e. Serotonergic and alpha receptors

71. A 42-year-old man on a short course of diazepam for generalised anxiety disorder has a memory problem. Usually, it would be:

   a. Retrograde amnesia

   b. Anterograde amnesia

   c. Anterograde and retrograde amnesia

   d. Procedural memory loss

   e. Sensory memory loss

72. Which one of these statements about MAOIs is correct?

   a. Clorgiline is a selective MAO-B inhibitor

   b. MAO-B platelet activity can be measured directly

   c. Tyramine is metabolised more in the liver than intestine

   d. Long term treatment with MAOIs causes down regulation of 5-HT-1A receptor

e. MAOIs cause a rebound increase in stage 4 sleep after discontinuation of treatment

73. Which one of these statements about tricyclic antidepressants is correct?
    a. Long term use leads to increase in D1 receptors
    b. They cause miosis by inhibiting cholinergic function
    c. They increase latency of onset of REM sleep
    d. Amitriptyline increases its own absorption
    e. They cause atropine psychosis due to peripheral muscarinic activity

74. Which one of these statements about SSRIs is correct?
    a. Paroxetine is the most potent of the SSRIs
    b. Citalopram is the least selective of the SSRIs
    c. SSRIs are slowly and incompletely absorbed from the gut
    d. SSRIs increase carbohydrate craving
    e. SSRIs are cytochrome inducers

75. Which one of the following is not a result of alpha-1 receptor blockade by trazodone?
    a. Orthostatic hypotension
    b. Nasal congestion
    c. Impaired ejaculation
    d. Priapism
    e. Mydriasis

76. The following characteristics will favour a good outcome in lithium treatment for bipolar affective disorder except:
    a. Having mood-incongruent psychotic symptoms
    b. Bipolar Type 1 Disorder
    c. Course of illness with a sequence of mania followed by depression
    d. Neuroticism
    e. Obsessionality

77. MAO-B acts on all the following, except:

a. Dopamine

b. Noradrenaline

c. Tyramine

d. Phenylethylamine

e. Benzylamine

78. The following are due to amitriptyline's activity on peripheral muscarinic receptors, except:

a. Pyrexia

b. Dry mouth

c. Glaucoma

d. Constipation

e. Urinary retention

79. Which one of these is an imidazopyridine hypnotic?

a. Zopiclone

b. Zolpidem

c. Zaleplon

d. Temazepam

e. Nitrazepam

80. Which one of these is an antiepileptic medication that acts by inhibiting GABA transaminase?

a. Gabapentin

b. Lamotrigine

c. Tiagabine

d. Vigabatrin

e. Sodium valproate

81. Following ECT there is a reduction in:

a. Noradrenaline

b. Serotonin

c. Dopamine

d. GABA

e. Acetylcholine

82. Mr Darns has recently found that strangers on the street are smiling at him and he has found it difficult to eat alongside his colleagues at work. What is his condition called?

a. Specific phobia

b. Schizoid personality disorder

c. Social phobia

d. Panic disorder

e. Adjustment disorder

83. Vicki, a petite girl, weighs 5 stone 4 pounds and eats a bowl of cereal a day. She finds her body unattractive and fat, and exercises at the gym for six hours every day. She feels very low because of her body image and has tried to harm herself in the past. What is her condition called?

a. Bulimia nervosa

b. Anorexia nervosa

c. Depression with somatic symptoms

d. Eating disorder not otherwise specified (NOS)

e. Hyperthyroidism

84. Mr Kane comes from a dysfunctional family. His mother is an odd lady, very strong and powerful, whereas his dad keeps to himself and is very passive. Mr Kane develops schizophrenia. A plausible explanation is:

a. Refrigerator mother

b. Marital schism

c. Marital skew

d. Double bind

e. Expressed emotion

85. Mr Somes presents to the GP with a 10-month history of sweating, tremor, palpitation and precordial persistent pain. He has been excessively investigated and seen by a cardiologist, and there is no evidence of IHD. Nevertheless he continues to believe that he has a serious heart condition. What is his actual condition called?

   a. Binswanger's disease

   b. Somatisation

   c. Generalised anxiety disorder

   d. Hypochondriasis

   e. Somatoform autonomic dysfunction

86. Mr Jones, a banker in the City, obtains gratification by rubbing against women travelling on the crowded Dockland Railways. What is this condition called?

   a. Frotteurism

   b. Fetishism

   c. Exhibitionism

   d. Voyeurism

   e. Masochism

87. Jane presents with darkened skin over the metacarpo-phalangeal joints of her second and third fingers. What is this condition called?

   a. Omega sign

   b. Chvostek's sign

   c. Kernig's sign

   d. Russell's sign

   e. Hoffmann's sign

88. Twenty-two-year-old Mr Winston presents with depression, fatigue and weight loss, difficulties with attention and concentration and darkness of the exposed areas of his body. This condition is called:

   a. Hypothyroidism

   b. Hypopituitarism

c. Addison's disease

d. Cushing's disease

e. Major depressive disorder

89. Mr Taylor has been diagnosed with a delusional disorder. On further exploration, it turns out that he has been a man who never trusted anyone and has been self-righteous all his life. It is easy to get on his wrong side and he has been losing friendships because simple actions made him feel threatened and deceived. What is the name of his condition?

a. Paranoid schizophrenia

b. Schizotypal disorder

c. Paranoid personality disorder

d. Narcissistic personality disorder

e. Schizoid personality disorder

90. A university student spends brief periods sleeping day and night. This condition is known as:

a. Psychomotor retarded depression

b. Klein-Levin syndrome

c. Pickwickian syndrome

d. Narcolepsy

e. Somnambulism

91. A Sri Lankan man presents with fear, depression and fatigue, and attributes it to excessive masturbation and losing semen. What is the name of his condition?

a. Dhat

b. Koro

c. Latah

d. Piblokto

e. Susto

92. Mr Madina presents with a 12-month history of memory impairment and language dysfunction. Characteristic pathological features that might be present include all, except:

    a. Neuritic plaques

    b. Reactive astrocytosis

    c. Lewy bodies

    d. Hirano bodies

    e. Amyloid angiopathy

93. Mr Ryder presents to A&E with a history of depression. Objective evidence of his mood can be inferred from:

    a. Motor activity

    b. Facial expressions

    c. Behaviour during the interview

    d. Patient's stated feeling

    e. Speech

94. Mrs Ayres has been diagnosed with schizophrenia and is worried about the possibility of her children developing schizophrenia. The risk of schizophrenia increases in:

    a. Identical twins

    b. Persons adopted at birth by a schizophrenic mother

    c. Cigarette smokers

    d. Persons conceived during summer

    e. Persons experiencing a birth injury

95. Mrs Jenner has recently lost her husband after his protracted fight with prostate cancer. Which of the following is indicative of a pathological grief reaction?

    a. Denial

    b. Clearing his room

    c. Visual hallucination

    d. Signing up for counselling

    e. Joining a charity for fighting prostate cancer

96. Significant memory impairment is caused by lesions in the:
    a. Anterior perforated substance
    b. Hippocampus
    c. Mamillary bodies
    d. Dorso-medial nucleus of thalamus
    e. Uncus

97. Mr Brendon has been diagnosed with compensation neurosis. What is true in relation to compensation neurosis?
    a. Improvements tend to occur after financial settlement
    b. Severe difficulties with sleep
    c. Seeking financial compensation after sustaining a relatively major injury
    d. Return to work is unusual
    e. Absence of frontal headaches

98. Mr Gomer has auditory hallucinations in clear consciousness. This could be caused by:
    a. Amphetamine abuse
    b. Atropine poisoning
    c. Mushroom poisoning
    d. Alcohol withdrawal
    e. Delirium

99. Which one of these statements is true regarding the classification of psychiatric disorders?
    a. Most diagnoses are dependent on one core symptom
    b. Symptoms used to identify disorders can be reliably elicited
    c. ICD-10 is theoretical
    d. DSM-IV is theoretical
    e. Diagnosis obtained using psychodynamic formulation is the most reliable

100. Mr Schwimmer is admitted under Section 3 to an acute psychiatric unit. When a trainee interviews him on his first day he finds it difficult to disclose his thoughts. Which of the following behaviours of the trainee could cause this?

   a. Normalisation

   b. Premature reassurance

   c. Appropriate open and closed questions

   d. Switching

   e. Agenda setting

101. Mrs Saunders lost her husband three weeks ago. How would you clinically differentiate between morbid and normal grief?

   a. Persistent denial of loss

   b. Auditory hallucination

   c. Recurrent nightmares involving the deceased

   d. Searching behaviour

   e. Self-blame

102. Which one of these is a bicyclic compound?

   a. Fluoxetine

   b. Fluvoxamine

   c. Mianserin

   d. Bupropion

   e. Trazodone

103. The primary metabolic pathway involved in the elimination of MAOIs is:

   a. Deamination

   b. Oxidation

   c. Hydroxylation

   d. Acetylation

   e. Reduction

104. Which one of these statements about MAOIs is correct?

  a. Irreversible MAOIs are more suitable for treating moderate rather than severe depression

  b. TCAs are more effective than MAOIs in the presence of anxiety with depression

  c. Imipramine is more effective than MAOIs if hypochondriacal symptoms are present along with anxiety

  d. MAOIs are suitable for treatment of simple, social and agoraphobias

  e. MAOIs are useful in treating obsessive-compulsive disorder (OCD) in the absence of phobias

105. A specific indication for use of moclobemide is:

  a. Agoraphobia

  b. Simple phobia

  c. Social phobia

  d. OCD with hypochondriacal symptoms

  e. Bulimia nervosa

106. SSRIs down-regulate all the following receptors except:

  a. 5-HT-1A

  b. 5-HT-2

  c. Beta-2

  d. D-1

  e. GABA

107. Mrs Johnson says that she has been on an antidepressant medication that caused extrapyramidal side-effects (EPSE). Which of these medications is it?

  a. Amitriptyline

  b. Imipramine

  c. Lofepramine

  d. Dothiepin

  e. Amoxapine

108. Linda has been diagnosed with Briquet's syndrome. The medication that has evidence supporting its use in this condition is:

   a. Trazodone

   b. Venlafaxine

   c. Mirtazapine

   d. Escitalopram

   e. Amitriptyline

109. Mrs Waller could develop atropine psychosis on which of these medications:

   a. Imipramine

   b. Desipramine

   c. Trazodone

   d. Nefazadone

   e. Fluoxetine

110. Eight-year-old Will develops enuresis. A treatment option is:

   a. Nortriptyline

   b. Amitriptyline

   c. Desipramine

   d. Clomipramine

   e. Paroxetine

111. A tricyclic that is unlikely to provoke an attack of glaucoma is:

   a. Clomipramine

   b. Lofepramine

   c. Dothiepin

   d. Amitriptyline

   e. Imipramine

112. A 49-year-old man presents with confusion, distended abdomen and absent bowel sounds since being treated for depression. The most likely causal agent is:

   a. Fluvoxamine

   b. Amitriptyline

   c. Mirtazapine

d. Trazodone

e. Venlafaxine

113. Mr Kensington develops septicaemia and an FBC shows agranulocytosis following antidepressant treatment. The potential causal drug is:

a. Viloxazine

b. Nomifensine

c. Maprotiline

d. Nortriptyline

e. Moclobemide

114. Unlike other SSRIs, sertraline is primarily metabolised by:

a. Hydroxylation

b. Deamination

c. Oxidation

d. Demethylation

e. Acetylation

115. A 72-year-old lady is observed to have papilloedema and bilateral extensor plantar reflexes along with cognitive impairment. What is her condition?

a. Multiple sclerosis

b. Guillain Barré syndrome

c. Polyarteritis nodosa

d. Chronic subdural haematoma

e. CADASIL (cerebral autosomal dominant arteriopathy with subcortical infarcts and leucoencephalopathy)

116. Mutations in the cystatin gene are associated with:

a. CADASIL

b. ANCA-polyarteritis nodosa

c. Hereditary cerebral haemorrhage Icelandic type

d. Amyotrophic lateral sclerosis

e. Pick's disease

117. A history of insomnia and thalamic dementia indicates:
    a. Amyotrophic lateral sclerosis
    b. Fatal familial insomnia
    c. Kleine-Levin syndrome
    d. Gerstmann-Straussler syndrome
    e. Whipple's disease

118. The following disorders are commonly associated with depression, except:
    a. Apathetic hyperthyroidism
    b. Addison's disease
    c. Primary hyperparathyroidism
    d. Hypercalcaemia
    e. Hypothyroidism

119. Mrs Smith experienced the loss of her husband six months ago. She continued bingo and cathedral groups in a very resilient way, but recently she's had pervasive guilt and suicidal thoughts. What is her condition?
    a. Bereavement
    b. Depression
    c. Delusional disorder
    d. Paraphrenia
    e. Dementia

120. Mrs Levy, 77 years old, had been diagnosed with depression. Which of the following is true in this scenario?
    a. EEG will show increased total REM sleep and REM latency
    b. Latency in evoked cortical potentials is equal between depression and control groups
    c. Focal abnormalities in cerebral blood flow are seen with PET
    d. The risk of depression in the first-degree relatives of late-onset depression is 20%
    e. All the above

121. Which one of the following is not true regarding the prognosis of depression in the elderly?

   a. 90% of successful suicides have a clear-cut history of depression

   b. Relapse is most likely in first 18 months to 2 years after an initial episode

   c. Studies have not shown that elderly depressive patients do better than younger individuals

   d. Duration of symptoms of more than 2 years is a poor prognostic factor

   e. Approximately two-thirds of elderly patients who attempt suicide have a psychiatric disorder

122. Which of the following is true regarding mania in the elderly?

   a. The average age of onset is 55 years

   b. Female to male ratio is 1:1

   c. One-year community incidence is 0.1%

   d. Mania is present in 12% of in-patient affective patients

   e. Right-sided lesions in the brain are associated with mania

123. Factors associated with late paraphrenia include all the following except:

   a. Female gender

   b. Hearing loss

   c. Visual impairment

   d. Lack of family history

   e. Unmarried status

124. The following are advantages of MRI compared to CT, with the exception of:

   a. Distinguishes between temporal lobe and posterior lobe structures

   b. Gives a three-dimensional display of the brain

   c. Sensitive to white matter lesions

   d. Does not cause exposure to ionising radiation

   e. Calcified lesions are poorly visualised

125. Which one of these is a depot preparation that takes about 2–18 hours to peak level in plasma?

a. Fluphenazine decanoate

b. Pipothiazine palmitate

c. Flupenthixol decanoate

d. Clopenthixol decanoate

e. Haloperidol decanoate

126. The following are clinical features of acute dystonia, except:

a. Supine arms

b. Adductor spasm

c. Plantar flexion-inversion

d. Lateral deviation of jaw

e. Anterocollis of neck

127. The following are non-drug variables influencing tardive dyskinesia, except:

a. Age

b. Gender

c. Previous EPSE

d. Age at onset of psychosis

e. Diabetes mellitus

128. Limb apraxia is caused by damage to the:

a. Left temporal lobe

b. Left parietal lobe

c. Right parietal lobe

d. Right temporal lobe

e. Right frontal lobe

129. Eye intorsion is served by the:

a. Optic nerve

b. Oculomotor nerve

c. Trochlear nerve

d. Trigeminal nerve

e. Abducens nerve

130. The earliest sign of papilloedema is:
    a. Blurring and heaping of nasal disc margin
    b. Blurring and heaping of temporal disc margin
    c. Pinkness of the disc
    d. Loss of spontaneous pulsation of retinal veins
    e. Engorgement and dilatation of the retinal vessels

131. Upper quadrantic field defects are caused by lesions in the:
    a. Optic chiasma
    b. Optic tract
    c. Optic radiation
    d. Temporal lobe
    e. Parietal lobe

132. A pupil fixed to light, but constricting on convergence is characteristic of:
    a. Syringomyelia
    b. Young women
    c. Neurosyphilis
    d. Pontine glioma
    e. Horner's syndrome

133. Failure of up-gaze and pupillary convergence reflex is seen in:
    a. Horner's syndrome
    b. Internuclear ophthalmoplegia
    c. Parinaud's syndrome
    d. Ramsay-Hunt syndrome
    e. Guillain Barré syndrome

134. A man presents with LMN facial weakness, failure of conjugate lateral gaze and contralateral hemiparesis. This is due to a lesion involving the facial nerve at which level:
    a. Within the pons
    b. In the cerebellopontine angle
    c. Within the petrous temporal bone
    d. Within the face
    e. At the geniculate ganglion

135. A man presents with downbeat jerk nystagmus. This is seen most commonly in lesions of:
    a. Middle ear
    b. Cerebellum
    c. Spino-cerebellar tract
    d. Foramen magnum
    e. All the above

136. Which one of these statements about endocrine disorders is correct?
    a. A higher incidence of depression is reported in Cushing's from adrenal rather than pituitary disease
    b. In contrast to Cushing's syndrome, steroid treatment is most commonly associated with mild elation of mood
    c. Delirium associated with low calcium levels is termed parathyroid crisis
    d. Secondary hypoparathyroidism presents with intellectual impairment
    e. Depression in phaeochromocytoma responds to ECT

Paper 2

1. Two-year-old John is shown a model of three mountains positioned side by side, each with a distinctive summit. He is asked to select from a collection of photos a picture showing what this array would look like to another person sitting at the opposite side of this model. Which statement is true?

   a. The child is egocentric because id and superego balance out each other

   b. A child in the sensorimotor stage will successfully complete this task

   c. A preoperational stage child will show the mountains in left-right reversal

   d. A two-year-old child will show its own view

   e. This is a test in the concrete operational stage

2. Non-conservation is seen at which age(s)?

   a. 7 years

   b. 8 years

   c. 9 years

   d. 10 years

   e. All the above

3. Reinforcer is a term used in which of the following?

   a. Classical conditioning

   b. Operant conditioning

   c. Punishment

   d. Social learning

   e. Deductive learning

4. Extinction is used in all except which of the following?

   a. Massing

   b. Flooding

   c. Implosion theory

   d. Blocking

   e. Systematic desensitisation

5. Forgetting is exhibited by deep-sea divers when they read lists of words either on-shore or underwater. Which of the following is true?

   a. This phenomenon is similar to that when learning whilst smoking cannabis

   b. This phenomenon is state dependent learning

   c. Forgetting is due to interference

   d. This phenomenon is an experiment to demonstrate the effect of attention

   e. This phenomenon is an experiment to demonstrate context dependent memory

6. Which is true?

   a. Computer simulations of memory use stage models

   b. Stage model of recall is associated with McClelland

   c. SAM is Script Activated Mechanism

   d. ACT is based on theories of declarative, semantic and procedural memories

   e. None of the above

7. A man with a desire to touch women in a crowded tube keeps this impulse under control by imagining that he will be arrested and imprisoned for such a sexual offence. The phenomenon is:

   a. Discrimination

   b. Aversive conditioning

   c. Covert sensitisation

   d. Escape conditioning

   e. Punishment

8. Choose the true definition:
   a. Semantics – the study of meaning of language
   b. Phonology – the study of basic sounds of a particular language
   c. Pragmatics – the study of how we use language
   d. Syntax – the rules whereby words are ordered to form sentences
   e. All of the above

9. All the following are true, except:
   a. The Verbal subset of WAIS-R consists of six subtests
   b. The WMS-R has nine items
   c. The HRNB has ten items
   d. The Rennick Repeatable Battery has seven items
   e. The Stroop Colour–Word Interference Test has three components

10. The following apply to scoring in Luria-Nebraska Neuropsychological Battery:
    a. 0 is normal
    b. 1 is probably organic
    c. 2 is definitely organic
    d. All the above
    e. B and C are true

11. Which one of these statements about emotion is correct?
    a. According to Freud, emotion is seen as a noxious state that compels ameliorative action
    b. Emotion is an unconditioned response that results from previous learning
    c. Emotion is a state of inactivation compelled by survival-related activities
    d. Emotion is less intense than mood
    e. Emotion is self-perpetuating

12. Which one of these statements about appraisal is correct?

    a. It emerged through research on war neuroses

    b. Primary appraisal concerns options or prospects for managing a given encounter

    c. Secondary appraisal signifies what is important or significant to the person

    d. Two forms of appraisal act independently

    e. It is the basis of the 'non-functional theory' of emotion

13. Which one of these statements about emotional processing is correct?

    a. Systems principle – emotions are products of two separate process and structure principles

    b. Developmental principle – emotion is an ever-changing phenomenon involving a configuration of a large number of variables

    c. Lazarus outlined the process-oriented approach and postulated five principles

    d. Specificity principle – each emotion is defined by a unique and specific relationship between person and environment

    e. Developmental principle – individual emotions can be understood in reference to particular patterns of appraisal that emerge over the course of the given encounter

14. Which one of these statements about functions of social support is correct?

    a. Robert Weiss outlines five relational provisions that an adequate social life should make available

    b. Esteem support is the same as emotional support

    c. Social companionship provides direct assistance, such as help with housework

    d. Motivational support is supported by research evidence

    e. Instrumental support involves the provision of information, advice and guidance

15. Which one of these statements about social support is correct?

a. People who participate in a broad range of domains have shallower mental health than those who confine themselves to one or two domains

b. Density of a support network is related to teenage pregnancy

c. Finding work outside the home protects against anxiety disorders

d. Perceived adequacy of support is a minor predictor of mental health

e. All are true

16. Which one of these statements about expressed emotion is correct?

a. Emotional involvement is a factor in predicting schizophrenia

b. More than 35 hours of contact with relatives was a better predictor of relapse than non-compliance with medication

c. Level of hostility is an important factor in the relapse of depression

d. Apparently superficial contact and conversation has little research evidence in support of preventing relapse

e. Expressed emotion was studied by Brown and Harris

17. Which one of these statements about family is correct?

a. People who have never married have better physical health than those who are married

b. Divorced and widowed people have lowest mental health

c. Cohesion relates autonomy of family members as individuals

d. Connected and disengaged are types of adaptability

e. Rigid and flexible are types of cohesion

18. Which one of these definitions of family types is correct?
    a. Mr Smith and Mr Smith, twin brothers, share unequal power – optimal family
    b. In Mr Smith's family, rule changes are implicit – optimal family
    c. Mrs Smith, an unemployed widow, always claims that help is on its way – triangulation
    d. Mr Smith and his son are engulfed by family roles and lack autonomy – enmeshed family
    e. Mr Smith is close to his son, but distant from his daughter – disengaged family

19. The following are true regarding self-concept, except:
    a. Maslow – growth motivation
    b. Kelly – reinterpreting personal construct
    c. Bandura – efficacy expectation
    d. Rogers – unconditional positive regard
    e. All of the above

20. Which of the following is a test used in determining pre-morbid intelligence of a 70-year-old coal miner?
    a. NART
    b. WAIS-R
    c. Rey-Osterrieth Complex figure
    d. MMPI
    e. None of the above

21. Which one of the following is a test used in primary schools for the assessment of graphomotor ability?
    a. WAIS-R
    b. Motor quotient
    c. Ray-Osterrieth complex figure
    d. Drawing test
    e. Gross motor skill

22. The cut-off for which particular subset is lowest when compared to other areas of development?

   a. Sensory quotient

   b. Intelligence quotient

   c. Motor quotient

   d. Language development

   e. Visual milestones

23. HRNB includes all except which of the following?

   a. MMPI

   b. WAIS-R

   c. Trail making test

   d. Stroop Colour–Word Interference Test

   e. Category Test

24. A psychiatrist from a developing country presents the case of a 21-year-old male by video link at RCPsych Annual Conference. Despite being told by his psychiatrist to resist being pushed, when merely touched on his back the man propels on to the wall. This phenomenon is:

   a. Mitgehen

   b. Gegenhalten

   c. Witzelsucht

   d. Vorbeigehen

   e. Verstimmung

25. A 22-year-old man, seen for first time by a psychiatrist, is very perplexed and claims that he could feel something bad happening around him. This phenomenon is:

   a. Verstimmung

   b. Gedankenlautwerden

   c. Mitmachen

   d. Vorbeigehen

   e. Wahnstimmung

26. A 72-year-old male admitted to EMAU, when asked what the month was, said 'April' and when asked what the year was, said 'April'. This condition is known as:

a. Echolalia

b. Palilalia

c. Paraphasia

d. Perseveration

e. Verbigeration

27. A 29-year-old man with a past history of schizophrenia, claims that his hand becomes numb as soon as he switches on his newly bought LCD television. This condition is known as:

a. Functional hallucination

b. Kinaesthetic hallucination

c. Reflex hallucination

d. Somatic passivity

e. Elementary hallucination

28. When you get into the car on a drizzly, rainbow-lit sunny-sky day, you suddenly remember that you have been in this scene before. This is known as:

a. A memory disorder

b. Jamais vu

c. Déjà vu

d. A type of misidentifying paramnesia

e. Normality of affect

29. Mr Brown, who had functioned as a high-achieving banker all his life but is now suspected of having dementia, forgets a few things on his shopping list and reports that the supermarket does not stock these items. This known as:

a. Fantastic confabulation

b. Delusional misidentification

c. Confabulation of embarrassment

d. Social confabulation

e. Suggestibility

30. Which one of these statements is not true of perseveration?
    a. It is associated with disturbance of memory
    b. It is a sign of organic brain disease
    c. It is useful in differentiating from dissociative abnormalities
    d. It is a pathognomonic sign
    e. It is a response appropriate to first stimulus but inappropriate to second stimulus

31. In schizophrenia, there is a marked disturbance of:
    a. Primary memory
    b. Working memory
    c. Procedural memory
    d. Episodic memory
    e. Semantic memory

32. Regarding the Ganser state, all the following features are true, except:
    a. Recent history of typhus
    b. Hallucinations
    c. Amnesia for the duration of symptoms
    d. Clouding of consciousness with orientation retained
    e. Hysterical stigmata

33. All the following are phases of development according to Freud, except:
    a. Oral
    b. Anal
    c. Phallic
    d. Oedipal
    e. Genital

34. According to Jung, all the following are archetypes, except:

a. Anima

b. Shadow

c. Persona

d. Old woman

e. Self

35. Which one of these defence mechanisms is used by an infant in a paranoid-schizoid stage?

a. Projection

b. Splitting

c. Displacement

d. Regression

e. Suppression

36. Melanie Klein is associated with:

a. Depressive position

b. Paranoid position

c. Penis envy

d. Sadism

e. Castration

37. The squiggle game is associated with:

a. Klein

b. Winnicott

c. Fairburn

d. Anna Freud

e. Ainsworth

38. A woman experienced pain whenever certain words were said. This condition is known as:

a. Functional hallucination

b. Reflex hallucination

c. Haptic hallucination

    d. Visceral hallucination

    e. Hypochondriasis

39. All the following are true regarding sensory deprivation, except:
    a. Inability to tolerate the situation
    b. It is patternless and meaningless
    c. It produces intellectual impairment
    d. It can be measured using galvanic skin response
    e. It can produce perceptual changes

40. False beliefs include all, except:
    a. Primary delusions
    b. Secondary delusions
    c. Sensitive ideas of reference
    d. Obsessions
    e. Overvalued ideas

41. Kendlar's dimensions of delusion include all, except:
    a. Extension
    b. Pressure
    c. Intuition
    d. Extension
    e. Disorganisation

42. The concept of autochthonous idea was formulated by:
    a. Jaspers
    b. Gruhle
    c. Wernicke
    d. Kurt Schneider
    e. Carl Schneider

43. The following are primary delusions, except:
    a. Delusional intuition
    b. Delusional misinterpretation
    c. Delusional memory
    d. Delusional atmosphere
    e. Delusional percept

44. Which one of these statements about intrinsic motivation theory is correct?
    a. High arousal leads to an optimum degree of alertness
    b. The subject requires a high level of arousal to attain a high level of performance
    c. It includes need to achieve (nAch)
    d. It is associated with cognitive assonance
    e. It is associated with aptitude-discrepant behaviour

45. Which one of these statements about theories of emotion is correct?
    a. Experience of emotion is primarily a somatic response to the perception of events
    b. James and Lange worked together to develop a theory of emotion
    c. According to the Cannon-Bard theory, signals are relayed from the cerebral cortex to the thalamus
    d. Bard performed an experiment in which subjects were injected with adrenaline
    e. Schacter's cognitive labelling theory says that conscious experience of an emotion is a function of the stimulus, somatic responses, and cognitive factors

46. All the following pairings are true, except:
    a. Contact comfort – Harlow
    b. Imprinting – Lorenzo
    c. Attachment – Bowlby

d. Paranoid position – Anna Freud

e. Object relations – Winnicott

47. Which one of these statements about separation from mother is correct?
    a. First phase is despair
    b. First phase is attachment
    c. Second phase is protest
    d. Second phase is detachment
    e. Manifestation of protest involves searching behaviour

48. Which one of these features is not characteristic of the dysfunctional Simpson family?
    a. Overprotection
    b. Ambiguous communication
    c. Myths
    d. Isolation
    e. Enmeshment

49. Childhood sexual abuse leads to all, except:
    a. Bipolar affective disorder
    b. Dissociative disorder
    c. Borderline personality disorder
    d. Increased incidence of homosexuality
    e. Eating disorder

50. Physical abuse in childhood leads to all, except:
    a. Nightmares
    b. Paranoia
    c. Splitting
    d. Drug and alcohol dependence
    e. Delayed language development

51. Which one of these statements about IQ is correct?

    a. Organic psychosyndromes reduce the verbal score more than the performance score

    b. The verbal scale is influenced by social cultural factors more than the performance scale

    c. IQ is stable in healthy people after 6 years

    d. Moderate mental retardation IQ is 50–69

    e. Creativity requires convergent thinking

52. Which one of these statements about insight is correct?

    a. It is unidimensional

    b. It is independent of the cultural factors

    c. ITAQ is an 11-item structured interview with score range of 0–22

    d. There is an inverse relation between insight, severity of pathology and positive affective disturbance

    e. Depressed patients have less insight than manic patients

53. Koro is:

    a. Autoscopy

    b. Somatisation

    c. Derealisation

    d. Desomatisation

    e. Heautoscopy

54. A 29-year-old schoolteacher presents with a 6-year history of pain involving the left side of the body. There is no physiological evidence for such pain. What is this condition?

    a. Somatisation disorder

    b. Persistent somatoform pain disorder

    c. Hypochondriasis

    d. Somatoform autonomic dysfunction

    e. Body dysmorphic disorder

55. Astasia-abasia is:

   a. A dissociative disorder
   b. Malingering
   c. A factitious disorder
   d. Somatisation
   e. Hypochondriasis

56. All the following are true regarding shop-lifting, except:

   a. More than three-fourths involve women
   b. One-third of shoplifters are under the age of 18
   c. 33% suffer from neuroses
   d. 17% have a personality disorder
   e. Fisher classified kleptomania into five categories

57. John, a 14-year-old boy who had to endure the divorce of his parents, develops forced vocalisations taking the form of obscene words or phrases. This phenomenon is:

   a. Echolalia
   b. Logoclonia
   c. Echopraxia
   d. Coprolalia
   e. Coprophagia

58. Mr Pembroke had always been someone who faced the world from a position of submission and humiliation. This personality disorder is known as:

   a. Dependent
   b. Narcissistic
   c. Anxious
   d. Paranoid
   e. Emotionally unstable

59. Mr Brown's body can be put into any posture despite him being asked to resist such movements. All the following are true regarding this symptom, except:

a. It is called mitmachen

b. Kahlbaum was the first person to describe this

c. The German equivalent is mitmachen

d. Mitgehen is one variant of this

e. Psychological pillow is another name for this behaviour

60. The following are defence mechanisms used in OCD, except:

a. Isolation

b. Undoing

c. Reaction formation

d. Repression

e. Intellectualisation

61. A 62-year-old-man relapsed into schizophrenia after a period of 18 years and preferred to be started on haloperidol. Which statement is true regarding clinical management?

a. The predominant sign of drug-induced Parkinsonism is rigidity

b. An increase in dose of the antipsychotic will alleviate symptoms of tardive dyskinesia in the short term

c. Oculogyric crisis will occur after 4 weeks

d. Akathisia will always respond to anticholinergic drugs

e. All the above are true

62. A 22-year-old man with schizophrenia is started on a thieno-benzodiazepine. Which of the following medications is of this type?

a. Quetiapine

b. Olanzapine

c. Piperazine

d. Clozapine

e. Fluphenazine

63. A 32-year-old man develops bon-bon sign with antipsychotics. This sign is seen in:

a. Neuroleptic malignant syndrome

b. Akathisia

c. Tardive dyskinesia

d. Acute dystonia

e. Parkinsonism

64. Mrs Johnson was started on a mood stabiliser when she was diagnosed with bipolar affective disorder type 2. Her psychiatrist says that she needs to be dose titrated as this mood stabiliser induces its own metabolism. Which one is she taking?

a. Lithium

b. Carbamazepine

c. Sodium valproate

d. Semisodium valproate

e. Lamotrigine

65. A lady admitted to the acute ward with a relapse of bipolar affective disorder is started on lamotrigine in addition to another mood stabiliser she is already on. The pharmacist is concerned that this mood stabiliser will increase the possibility of lamotrigine toxicity. Which mood stabiliser is she already on?

a. Olanzapine

b. Lithium

c. Carbamazepine

d. Quetiapine

e. Topiramate

66. A 49-year-old-lady is been on antidepressant medication for more than 8 years. She has developed pins and needles and a burning type of pain on her feet and legs. Which antidepressant medication is she likely to be taking?

   a. Trazodone

   b. Imipramine

   c. Fluvoxamine

   d. Phenelzine

   e. Maprotiline

67. Mrs Saunders' ECG shows sinus tachycardia after she was commenced on a psychotropic for generalised anxiety disorder. The psychotropic could be:

   a. Chlordiazepoxide

   b. Lorazepam

   c. Alprazolam

   d. Buspirone

   e. Propranolol

68. A major site for lithium absorption is the:

   a. Stomach, when the pH is high

   b. Stomach, when the pH is low

   c. Small intestine, by active transport

   d. Small intestine, by passive transport

   e. Large intestine, where the water content is lower

69. Mrs Waller has been started on a hypnotic medication following admission for a severe depressive episode. Since starting the medication, she complains of a metallic taste on her tongue. The medication is most likely to be:

   a. Temazepam

   b. Nitrazepam

   c. Zopiclone

   d. Zolpidem

   e. Oxazepam

70. Mr Eriksson develops priapism on trazodone. This is due to:

    a. Alpha-1 agonism

    b. Beta-1 agonism

    c. Alpha-2 agonism

    d. Alpha-2 antagonism

    e. Alpha-1 antagonism

71. Which among the following statements is true with regard to adverse consequences from being on lithium treatment:

    a. One in four develop histological abnormalities of the kidneys

    b. A 20-times greater chance than the normal population of giving birth to a baby with Epstein's anomaly

    c. Compared to serum, breast milk has a 75% higher concentration of lithium

    d. Less than 25% develop T-wave inversion and flattening on their ECG

    e. Coarse tremor is common in mild toxicity

72. A 32-year-old lady is concerned about the thinning of her hairline since being on a mood stabiliser. Which mood stabiliser is it likely to be?

    a. Carbamazepine

    b. Lithium citrate

    c. Lithium carbonate

    d. Sodium valproate

    e. Lamotrigine

73. Mrs Stone is on phenelzine and she requires a mood stabiliser due to a revision of her diagnosis to bipolar disorder. Which mood stabiliser is contraindicated for her use?

    a. Olanzapine

    b. Carbamazepine

    c. Lithium

    d. Lamotrigine

    e. Sodium valproate

74. The following changes are associated with ECT, except:

a. A fall in prolactin is the most common acute change

b. An increase in insulin in the acute phase

c. A reduction in the plasma concentration of noradrenaline

d. An increase in substance P

e. A reduction in 24-hour urinary 5-HIAA

75. Mr Robinson, a right-handed individual, whilst talking to you about consenting to ECT has many questions about side-effects. With regards to ECT, which among the following statements is incorrect?

a. Co-morbid stomach cancer is a poor prognostic sign

b. Memory impairment would be more possible if the dose is increased following a poor response

c. Hypertension is a common side-effect from ECT

d. Unilateral ECT to right hemisphere will cause a loss of memory effect

e. Psychomotor retardation is a poor prognostic sign

76. Which one of these foods or drinks is safe to use along with MAOIs:

a. Chianti

b. Pickled herring

c. Smoked herring

d. Milk

e. Broad-bean pods

77. Which of these 5-HT receptor types involves an ion-channel-mediated second messenger system?

a. 1A

b. 1B

c. 1C

d. 2

e. 3

78. Phencyclidine acts by blocking which of these receptor types?
   a. GABA
   b. 5-HT-2
   c. D5
   d. NMDA
   e. Central muscarinic

79. Olanzapine is metabolised by:
   a. CYP1A2
   b. CYP2C9
   c. CYP2C19
   d. CYP2D6
   e. CYP3A4

80. 5-HTT is targeted by:
   a. Methylphenidate
   b. Reboxetine
   c. Amitriptyline
   d. Fluoxetine
   e. Mirtazapine

81. A Malaysian man shows sudden excitement with marked violence and paranoia. This behaviour is characteristic of:
   a. Amok
   b. Latah
   c. Cathard
   d. Windigo
   e. Piblokto

82. Since giving birth to twins Miss Anniston has been very tearful, low-spirited and has been avoiding food. She spends the night awake, and for the last 2 weeks has found it difficult to breast-feed her babies and believes that her breasts are involuting. What is this condition called?

    a. Maternity blues

    b. Postpartum depression

    c. Postpartum psychosis

    d. Adjustment disorder

    e. Conversion disorder

83. Mrs Schindler presents with a first episode of depression and is started on an SSRI. Seven days later she is found to be overactive and sleepless, which lasts for about 5 days. The symptoms resolve when the SSRI is stopped. What disorder is this?

    a. Bipolar type 2 disorder

    b. Bipolar type 1 disorder

    c. Unipolar mania

    d. Mixed affective disorder

    e. Substance induced mood disorder

84. Mr Gates has spent most of his life researching about a time machine. He is unmarried and has poor communication skills. He has very interesting thoughts and theories about extraterrestrial species. What is the name of this condition?

    a. Schizoid personality disorder

    b. Cyclothymic personality

    c. Schizotypal personality disorder

    d. Paranoid personality disorder

    e. Paranoid schizophrenia

85. Mrs Jones presents with mild memory impairment and has a shuffling gait. She has a history of urinary incontinence and the MRI shows enlarged ventricles. What is the most likely diagnosis?

    a. Normal pressure hydrocephalus

b. Supraventricular gaze palsy

c. Dementia due to vitamin B12 deficiency

d. Vascular dementia

e. Binswanger's disease

86. Mr Keane presents with a labile affect. His family claim that he has had mood swings ranging from irritability to apathy. His GP has diagnosed peripheral neuropathy and hypertension. He has greasy skin, a huge jaw and has impaired glucose tolerance (IGT). What is the name of his condition?

a. Addison's disease

b. Cushing's disease

c. Hyperparathyroidism

d. Acromegaly

e. Hypothyroidism

87. Mr Pitt has a long history of alcohol dependence. He is noted to have spasticity of his limbs and is unable to walk. On MMSE, he scores 20 and the MRI shows demyelination of the corpus callosum. What is the name of his condition?

a. Marchiafava-Bignami Syndrome

b. Wernicke's encephalopathy

c. Korsakoff's psychosis

d. Alcohol dementia

e. Pick's disease

88. Wayne presents with recurrent rapid, flapping and violent involuntary movements, with normal muscle tone. The suspected lesion is most likely in the:

a. Caudate nucleus

b. Putamen

c. Subthalamus

d. Globus pallidus

e. Striatum

89. A 49-year-old-man who lives on the street, presents to A&E with depression. He also complains of diarrhoea. A physical examination shows glossitis and dry, excoriated skin. His blood tests are unremarkable. These features are due to a deficiency of:

   a. Niacin

   b. Riboflavin

   c. Cyanocobalamin

   d. Thiamine

   e. Pantothenic acid

90. Mrs Burgess suffers from bipolar affective disorder. Which of the following statements is true regarding her condition?

   a. Compared to her friend who has unipolar affective disorder, she would have less frequent episodes

   b. Combined rate of unipolar and bipolar disorder in her first degree relatives is significantly higher than that in relatives of her friend

   c. Unlike her illness, her friend is right in saying that her friend's illness is twice as common in women than men

   d. The risk of bipolar affective disorder is the same for men and women

   e. There is an increased risk of depression alone in her sister

91. In contrast to DSM, ICD10 has all the following features, except:

   a. Post-psychotic depression is included under schizophrenia

   b. It contains a robust classification of short psychotic disorders

   c. Schizotypal disorders are included under schizophrenia

   d. Dissocial personality disorder is classed as a diagnostic entity

   e. It specifies 6 months as a criterion for schizophrenia

92. Depersonalisation-derealisation syndrome is associated with all the following except:

   a. Phobias

   b. Sensory deprivations

c. Depression

d. Near-death experience

e. OCD

93. An abnormal EEG can be seen in all the following except:

a. Alcohol dependence

b. Antisocial personality disorder

c. Cerebral abscess

d. Narcolepsy

e. Benzodiazepine dependence

94. Interviewing techniques that help to establish a therapeutic relationship include all except which one of the following?

a. Offering free rein for the patient at the start of the interview to describe his/her symptoms

b. Recording striking remarks verbatim

c. Maintaining constant eye contact

d. Paraphrasing

e. Encouraging reflection

95. Pathological features of Alzheimer's disease include all except which one of the following?

a. Wide cerebral sulci

b. Reduced cholinergic neurons

c. Loss of neurones in the basal nucleus of Meynert

d. Amyloid plaques and tangles

e. Localised atrophy of the cerebral cortex

96. With regard to performing a mental state examination, all the following are true except:
    a. Inability to sit during an interview occurs in the absence of mental state
    b. Inability to sit in schizophrenia signifies an increased risk of suicide
    c. Poor recall of the Babcock sentence is a reliable indicator of the presence of organic brain disorder
    d. A depressed mood in a patient may be suggested by raised medial aspect of the eyebrow
    e. Pseudohallucinations are commonly seen in clouded consciousness

97. Absent knee and ankle jerks are characteristic of which one of the following conditions?
    a. Punch-drunk syndrome
    b. Parkinson's disease
    c. Multiple sclerosis
    d. Guillain Barré syndrome
    e. Alzheimer's disease

98. Regarding sick role behaviour, which of these statements is not true?
    a. It was first described by Parsons
    b. It is behaviour adopted by those who consider themselves to be ill
    c. It leads to expectation of normal social obligations
    d. It is an abnormal behaviour
    e. It is prolonged in children

99. Which one of these is considered a prion dementia?
    a. Gerstmann-Straussler syndrome
    b. Sjögren's syndrome
    c. Friedreich's ataxia
    d. Shy-Drager syndrome
    e. HIV dementia

100. Which one of the following is characteristic of a brain-stem lesion (in contrast to a cortical lesion)?

a. Dysphagia

b. Vertigo

c. Dysphasia

d. All of the above

e. None of the above

101. Andy presents with coprolalia and winking of the eye. This can be treated effectively with:

a. Fluoxetine

b. Paroxetine

c. Fluvoxamine

d. Sertraline

e. Citalopram

102. A 21-year-old lady admitted to an acute psychiatric unit under the MHA presents with nausea, vomiting, hyperthermia, autonomic instability and on blood testing shows normal CK. Specific treatment will include:

a. Tetrabenazine

b. Procyclidine

c. Cyproheptadine

d. Benzhexol

e. Metoclopramide

103. A lady taking phenytoin as an anticonvulsant has a sudden exacerbation of phenytoin side-effects after commencing anti-depressant treatment. A potential cause is:

a. Trazodone

b. Nefazadone

c. Mianserin

d. Maprotiline

e. Reboxetine

104. Long-term use of St. John's Wort leads to the down-regulation of which receptor?

a. 5-HT-1A

b. 5-HT-2

c. Alpha-1

d. Alpha-2

e. Beta-1

105. Which one of these statements about lithium is correct?

a. Lithium intoxication spares lithium clearance

b. Lithium excretion is independent of glomerular filtration

c. The slow-release form of lithium reduces its bioavailability

d. There is significant inter-personal variation in serum level 12 hours post-dose

e. Lithium is 955 bound to proteins

106. Which one of these statements about lithium is incorrect?

a. Short-term lithium treatment increases turnover of serotonin

b. Long-term treatment increases platelet reuptake of serotonin

c. Lithium induces a reduced turnover of noradrenaline

d. Lithium increases super-sensitivity of dopamine receptors after chronic treatment with haloperidol

e. Lithium inhibits noradrenaline-induced cAMP activity

107. Which one of the following is not predictive of Mr Benmar's outcome from lithium treatment?

a. Age

b. Family history of bipolar illness

c. Paranoid feature

d. High obsessionality

e. Social support

108. Which one of these statements about treating lithium toxicity is not true?

a. In severe sodium deficiency, lithium acts by inhibiting aldosterone

b. Following recovery, some patients may be left with permanent neurological deficits

c. Vomiting, diarrhoea and coarse tremor may appear at a serum lithium level of 1.3 mmol/L

d. Haemodialysis is indicated when serum lithium level is above 2 mmol/L

e. When renal function is unimpaired, increasing fluid intake would be sufficient

109. Which one of these statements about side-effects of lithium is correct:

a. Raised serum parathormone is not a true hyperparathyroidism

b. T-wave flattening on ECG is benign and reversible

c. Rapid-cycling mood swings may be associated with subclinical hyperthyroidism

d. Acneiform eruptions and exfoliative dermatitis occur very rarely

e. Leucocytosis caused by lithium can be of use in medical disorders associated with leucopenia

110. Mr Simmons, who is on a mood stabiliser, presents with diplopia, constipation and allergic rash, and on investigation shows hyponatraemia, abnormal LFTs and thrombocytopenia. The most likely cause is:

a. Lithium

b. Carbamazepine

c. Sodium valproate

d. Olanzapine

e. Lamotrigine

111. The following are neurochemical changes associated with ECT, except:
    a. Depletion of dopamine in the hypothalamus
    b. Increased post-synaptic functioning of 5-HT-1A receptors
    c. Changes to GABA-B receptors
    d. Elevation of intrathecal TRH
    e. Up-regulation of beta-adrenoceptors

112. Long-term memory for autobiographical events is called:
    a. Procedural memory
    b. Episodic memory
    c. Semantic memory
    d. Echoic memory
    e. Implicit memory

113. Mrs Bergman has depression, and the plan is for her to undergo ECT. The following are predictors of good response, except:
    a. Moderate depressive episode with somatic symptoms
    b. Severe depressive episode with somatic symptoms
    c. Psychomotor retardation
    d. Presence of delusions
    e. Anxiety

114. Which one of these statements about neuroimaging is correct?
    a. Apo E4 alleles are associated with greater volume loss in the amygdala compared to the frontal lobe
    b. White matter lesions associated with prolonged relaxation time are seen in Alzheimer's disease more than vascular dementia
    c. In early dementia, reduced rCBF is confined to parietal lobes on SPECT
    d. PET-CBF and metabolism are uncoupled in Alzheimer's disease
    e. N-acetylaspartate is reduced in Pick's disease

115. The reasons why medical patients are not referred to psychiatrists include all, except:

   a. There is a poor working relationship between physician and psychiatrist

   b. The significance of psychological issues is denied

   c. The patient fears the physician's emotions

   d. The physician considers the patient to be too ill physically

   e. The physician feels he or she does not know the patient well enough

116. Which one of the following is not a true characteristic of nursing home residents?

   a. Older age range

   b. More females than males

   c. Poor physical health

   d. Over a quarter have dementia

   e. Degenerative disorders are more common

117. The following are incorrect regarding MHA except:

   a. Section 135 – removing an individual from a public place

   b. Section 136 – removing an individual from home

   c. Section 58 – patient consenting to treatment, but not ECT

   d. National Assistance Act – to enforce abode, attendance for training and treatment, access to professionals

   e. Section 155 – to enter and inspect premises

118. 'Utterly unable to rejoice in anything . . . cannot comprehend, believe or think of anything that is comfortable.' This condition is known as:

   a. Alexithymia

   b. Anergy

   c. Apathy

   d. Anhedonia

   e. Amotivation

119. Loss of anticipatory pleasure and concern is known as:

a. Anhedonia

b. Anergy

c. Apathy

d. Alexithymia

e. Amotivation

120. The type of sleep disturbance traditionally associated with melancholia is:

a. Initial insomnia

b. Middle insomnia

c. Early-morning awakening

d. Hypersomnia

e. Daytime sleepiness

121. 'I am a worm and not a man.' A belief such as this is an example of:

a. Delusions of guilt

b. Thoughts of worthlessness

c. Hopelessness

d. Hypochondriasis

e. Nihilistic delusion

122. '. . . A sort of dead feeling, wooden inside, I've changed.' A statement such as this is an example of:

a. Autotopagnosia

b. Dysmorphophobia

c. Delusions of bodily change

d. Nihilistic delusion

e. Depersonalisation

123. La folie, a double form, is associated with:

a. Bleuler

b. Falret

c. Kraepelin

d. Leonhard

e. Baillarger

124. Acoustic neuroma is a lesion that affects the vestibular nerve at the level of the:

a. Cerebral cortex

b. Pons

c. Cerebellum

d. Cerebellopontine angle

e. Petrous temporal bone

125. Which one of the following spinal nerve–tendon reflex pairings is correct?

a. C4-C5 – supinator

b. C5-C6 – biceps

c. L4-L5 – knee

d. L4-L5 – ankle

e. None of the above

126. Which one of these statements about the parasympathetic supply to the bladder and genitalia is correct?

a. It is from S2-S4

b. It causes bladder wall contraction

c. It causes internal sphincter contraction

d. It causes erection of the penis

e. It causes engorgement of the clitoris

127. A 36-year-old-man presents with absent self-awareness, absent cyclical eye opening, a Glasgow Coma Scale score of E1-2, M1-4, V1-2 and polymorphic delta or theta waves on EEG. What state is he in?

a. Vegetative state

b. Locked-in-syndrome

c. Coma

d. Brain stem death

e. Delirium

128. The application of metrazol-induced seizure is associated with:

a. Meduna

b. Kretschmer

c. Cade

d. Charpentier

e. Kline

129. Which one of the following pairings is correct?

a. Systemic family therapy – Palazzoli

b. Structural family therapy – Minuchin

c. Interpersonal therapy – Klerman

d. Family therapy – Dicks

e. Biofeedback – Birk

130. Moreno is associated with:

a. Primal therapy

b. Psychobiology

c. Psychodrama

d. Therapeutic community

e. Transactional analysis

131. Reciprocal inhibition is associated with:

a. Wolpe

b. Braid

c. Sheldon

d. Harlow

e. Bill

132. Alexander is associated with:

a. Psychosomatic medicine

b. Dissociation

c. Moral insanity

d. Dysmorphophobia

e. Conolly

133. Faegerman is associated with:
a. Schizophreniform disorder
b. Psychogenic psychoses
c. Bouffée délirante
d. Atypical psychosis
e. Paranoia

134. According to Leonhard, thought disorder is prominent in:
a. Anxiety–happiness psychosis
b. Excited–inhibited confusion psychosis
c. Hyperkinetic–akinetic psychosis
d. Brief transient psychosis
e. All of the above

135. Which of these statements about sleep disorders is correct?
a. Subjects with insomnia rely on repression and denial
b. Obstructive sleep apnoea is also known as Gelineau's syndrome
c. The mode of inheritance of narcolepsy is dominant with complete penetrance
d. Menstrual hypersomnia usually occurs during the corpus phase
e. Pavor incubus (night terrors) occurs in 30% of children at least once

Paper 3

1. A child is shown four green counters and two blue counters, and asked whether there are more counters in total or more green counters. The child answers green. Which of the following is true?
   a. The child wrongly makes a transitive inference
   b. The child is in sensorimotor phase
   c. Lack of class inclusion is a part of concrete operational phase
   d. The child is 8 years of age
   e. The child is in the preoperational phase

2. According to Piaget, a child achieves the stage of adult cognition when the child:
   a. Is no longer egocentric
   b. Uses logical reasoning
   c. Is 16 years of age
   d. Succeeds in the pendulum test
   e. Enters the concrete operational phase

3. When comparing learned helplessness and depression, which of these statements is true?
   a. There is a similar time course of persistence
   b. Different levels of aggression are produced
   c. Cholinergic inactivation is produced in both
   d. Cognitive set does not change in both
   e. Both show increased levels of voluntary behaviour

4. The best screening tool for depression in 14–18-year-old adolescents is:

a. SCID

b. Child and Adolescent Assessment Scale

c. Becks Depression Inventory

d. Hamilton's Depression Rating Scale

e. Child Behaviour Checklist

5. Which one of the following is true, according to Chomsky?

a. Semantics is innate

b. Grammar is species specific

c. Semantics is species specific

d. Transformational grammar is required to understand sentences

e. Linguistic competence is the same as performance

6. A 39-year-old man played Lotto consistently every week with the hope of winning big one day. He has won small amounts of money on certain occasions. What is the reinforcement schedule demonstrated by his behaviour?

a. Variable ratio

b. Variable interval

c. Fixed ratio

d. Fixed interval

e. None of the above

7. Linguistic exchange to communicate for the sake of preserving communication is called:

a. Phonetic exchange

b. Phatic exchange

c. Exchange fallacy

d. Exchange of stock words

e. Stroke

8. An elderly man recovering in a surgical ward experiences fluctuating episodes of consciousness and visual hallucinations with altered sleep-wake cycle. The diagnosis is:
   a. Alzheimer's dementia
   b. Lewy Body disease
   c. Paraphrenia
   d. Acute psychotic episode
   e. Delirium

9. Which one of these statements about bonding is correct?
   a. Imprinting is reversible
   b. Bonding is primarily formation of attachment of infant to mother
   c. Klaus and Kennel proposed the hypothesis of bonding
   d. Bonding occurs only during the hours following birth
   e. There is a low incidence of physical abuse observed between mothers and low-birth-weight infants

10. Which one of these statements about developmental stages is correct?
    a. Adult levels of acuity are attained at 24 weeks
    b. Infants prefer simple stimuli, with low contrast
    c. Infants prefer to track face-type configurations from 12 weeks
    d. Infants prefer the mother's face when they are 12 weeks
    e. Infants do not have visual preferences

11. Which one of these statements about developmental stages is correct?
    a. Neonates show reflex facial expressions in response to a sweet taste
    b. Neonates prefer speech-type sounds
    c. Smiling becomes socially intent from 8 weeks
    d. Infants imitate facial expressions of others as they have an internal representation of self
    e. Neonates show attachment to strangers

12. Which one of these statements about developmental stages is correct?

   a. In turn-taking conversational modes, an infant always responds during pauses

   b. Reciprocal games emerge at 3 months

   c. The short face of the infant is meant to draw attention to its face

   d. Speech modifications made by care-givers towards infants are noticeable from birth to 2 years

   e. 'Motherese' is a form of speech shown by infants

13. Which one of these statements about attachment is correct?

   a. A hierarchy of attachment figures is formed

   b. Primary attachments may be formed through to early childhood

   c. The primary attachment figure is always the biological mother

   d. Attachment occurs because of a one-dimensional approach from infant to mother

   e. Attachment is an instant instinct

14. Which one of these statements about family and coping is correct?

   a. Minuchin hypothesised that family interactions play an important role in determining the prognosis of chronic illnesses

   b. Adaptive coping involves cognitive and social processes engaged in advance of a crisis

   c. Psychological denial is a method of coping

   d. Assimilative and adaptive methods are types of coping

   e. Reorganisation of family system is used in resistance coping

15. Which one of these statements about illness and illness behaviour is correct?

   a. Illness was defined by Parsons

   b. Exemption from normal social role is relative to nature of illness

c. Illness behaviour and death rate show a bimodal distribution in relationship to age

d. Abnormal illness behaviour is more common in women as opposed to men

e. Durkheim distinguished between different types of illness behaviour

16. A 39-year-old man working in a restaurant suffered a head injury. Following this, he developed an inability to set a table for dinner and to calculate the bill correctly, and he complained that he could not feel coins given as tip. Which area of his brain was damaged?

a. Left parietal lobe

b. Left temporal lobe

c. Bilateral parietal lobe

d. Bilateral temporal lobe

e. Parieto-occipital region

17. The practice of bowing to a leader, as practiced by African tribes, mirrors the action performed by animals whereby aggressive events are avoided. What is this known as?

a. Ritualisation

b. Social learning theory

c. Aggressive cue theory

d. Appeasement gesture

e. Origin of autism

18. In an attempt to reduce the yob culture of drunken adolescents, the Government decides to create a phobia for alcohol, but finds that it is more difficult than creating a phobia for snakes. This is due to:

a. Discrimination

b. Habituation

c. Incubation

d. Preparedness

e. Stimulus generalisation

19. In her psychotherapy session, Mrs Denver explained that her best way of dealing with difficulties was not to think about them. This is known as:

a. Suppression

b. Repression

c. Denial

d. Idealisation

e. Undoing

20. Mrs Singh, an immigrant from India, says that her adolescent son has been complaining of repetitive thoughts of harming her and that he has to utter a short mantra to prevent harm. This is known as:

a. Sublimation

b. Reaction formation

c. Undoing

d. Acting out

e. Rationalisation

21. Dr Smith, who always turns up late for work, claims that he would be in early if he were not stuck in traffic every day. This is known as:

a. Denial

b. Displacement

c. Projection

d. Rationalisation

e. Idealisation

22. Jamie, who has been a troublemaker and a yob, decided to take up a career in the army. This is known as:

a. Acting out

b. Displacement

c. Idealisation

d. Altruism

e. Sublimation

23. The following pairings are true, except:
  a. Schizophrenia – Kraepelin
  b. Catatonia – Kahlbaum
  c. Hebephrenia – Hecker
  d. Unitary psychosis – Griesinger
  e. Cycloid psychosis – Leonhard

24. Which one of these statements about psychopathology is incorrect?
  a. Observation is a type of descriptive psychopathology
  b. Psychopathology is systematic study of normal experience, cognition and behaviour
  c. Phenomenology is a type of descriptive psychopathology
  d. Descriptive psychopathology can be likened to conducting a medical history and examination
  e. Psychodynamics is an explanatory psychopathology model

25. Which one of these statements is incorrect?
  a. Descriptive psychopathology includes theoretical explanation for psychological events
  b. Phenomenology includes the study of both psychological and physical events
  c. Health according to the WHO includes concepts of the absence of disease or infirmity
  d. In typological abnormality, value, statistical and individual norms are abnormal
  e. Compared to descriptive psychopathology, in psychoanalytic psychopathology, no distinction is made between form and content

26. Which one of these statements about consciousness is correct?
    a. There are four dimensions of consciousness
    b. Consciousness is separable from the object of concentration
    c. Lucidity is related to vigilance
    d. In clouding of consciousness, though there is impaired awareness of the environment, perception and memory are retained
    e. Extreme enjoyment increases vigilance

27. Mr Smith, a 77-year-old gentleman admitted to the EMAU, is awake but drifts into sleep if left without any sensory stimulation. What stage of consciousness is he in?
    a. Clouding
    b. Drowsiness
    c. Sopor
    d. Coma
    e. Unconscious

28. Fluctuation in consciousness:
    a. Does not happen in epilepsy
    b. Occurs in healthy people
    c. Is very rarely associated with third ventricular tumours
    d. Decreases as the day progresses
    e. Reduces with mescaline

29. A 48-year-old woman who attends a Buddhist gathering describes a moment of sublime peace and a feeling of being one with all living species and nature. This is known as:
    a. Euphoria
    b. Ecstasy
    c. Elation
    d. Grandiosity
    e. Lability

30. Mr Smith, who is diagnosed with dysthymia, complains of inability to express his feelings and of having infrequent dreams. What condition does he have?

a. Dyslexia

b. Anhedonia

c. Alexithymia

d. Dysphoria

e. Apathy

31. A 49-year-old man with a diagnosis of negative schizophrenia appears to have no emotional reaction during his review in the Clozaril clinic. What is his condition known as?

a. Blunted affect

b. Flattened affect

c. Apathy

d. Dysthymia

e. Depression

32. A lawyer who is being treated for delirium tremens points to the other cubicles and says that they are jury stands and that the hospital is in fact the Old Bailey. What is his condition known as?

a. Pareidolia

b. Occupational delirium

c. Reduplicative paramnesia

d. Confabulation

e. Dysmegalopsia

33. Sixty-seven-year-old Mrs Wellington claims to see her relatives change temporarily into Beatles, both in external appearance and personality. What is her condition known as?

a. Intermetamorphosis delusion

b. Reverse subjective doubles syndrome

c. Autoscopy

d. Capgras' syndrome

e. De Clérambault's syndrome

34. Which one of these statements about personal time is correct?

   a. Personal time is objective

   b. The body clock runs a little faster

   c. The body clock is nearer to a 25-hour cycle

   d. When we extend the day, we prefer to do so in the early morning

   e. To extend the day, we prefer to make bed time later and the time we rise later

35. Which one of these statements about age disorientation is incorrect?

   a. It is a 10-year discrepancy between a patient's actual age and a patient's stated age

   b. It correlates with intellectual impairment in schizophrenia

   c. It is accompanied by underestimation of the duration of stay in hospital

   d. It is observed in patients with affective disorder

   e. It can be picked up on cognitive assessment using MMSE

36. Which one of these statements about affective disturbance of time is correct?

   a. In depression, real time seems to pass slowly as far as the patient is concerned

   b. Disturbance of time in affective disorders is related to depersonalisation

   c. In LSD intoxication, there is a sensation of living only in the future

   d. Giving up/given up complex is seen in endogenous depression

   e. Jamais vu is the sense of familiarity for objects that have been seen before

37. Which one of these statements about circadian rhythms is correct?

   a. Comparing internal time with clock time, there is a gradual decrease in estimated time

b. There is a greater overestimation of fixed intervals in the afternoon

c. The internal clock accelerates when the body temperature is raised

d. There is a phase advance of the sleep-wake cycle in depression

e. Travel from west to east is associated with depression

38. Which one of these statements about seasonal variation is correct?

a. There is a high rate of admission of patients with schizophrenia during spring months

b. Onset of depression and administration of ECT is common during autumn

c. There is a peak of admission of female manic patients in July

d. Compared to southern hemisphere, there is an excessive amount of birth dates for people with schizophrenia in winter months in the northern hemisphere

e. Suicide rates are lowest in the quarter containing April, May and June

39. 'Something funny is going on. I have been offered a whole world of new meanings.' This condition is known as:

a. Delusional percept

b. Delusional atmosphere

c. Delusional intuition

d. Delusional memory

e. Secondary delusion

40. According to Conrad, the five stages in delusion include all, except:

a. Trema

b. Apophany

c. Anastrophy

d. Encapsulation

e. Residuum

41. Which one of the following pairings is not correct?

   a. Delusions of persecution – Bleuler

   b. Sexual jealousy – Kraepelin

   c. Erotomania – Clérambault

   d. Delusional misidentification – Ellis

   e. Delusional infestation – Ekbom

42. Mrs Winnall falsely identifies her husband among strangers she sees in town. This condition is known as:

   a. Capgras' syndrome

   b. Syndrome of intermetamorphosis

   c. Syndrome of subjective doubles

   d. Prosopagnosia

   e. Fregoli's syndrome

43. Primary emotions classified by Plutchik include all, except:

   a. Anger

   b. Disgust

   c. Surprise

   d. Happiness

   e. Anticipation

44. Which one of these statements about communication is correct?

   a. Being an opinion leader is not a characteristic of being a persuasive communicator

   b. Message repetition is useful with high-intelligence people

   c. Two-sided communications are more effective with people of low intelligence

   d. Implicit messages are more persuasive for less intelligent people

   e. Interactive personal discussions are more persuasive than mass media communications

45. Which one of these statements about the sensorimotor stage is correct?

   a. Primary circular reaction occurs between 5 and 9 months

   b. Secondary circular reaction occurs from 1 year to 18 months

   c. The law of conservation is achieved at the end of the sensorimotor stage

   d. Object permanence is fully developed after approximately 18 months

   e. There are two types of circular reactions

46. All the following would apply to 6-year-old Abigail, except:

   a. Artificialism

   b. Creationism

   c. Egocentricity

   d. Object permanence

   e. Precausal reasoning

47. Which one of the following statements is true?

   a. Repetitive babbling occurs between 3 and 4 months

   b. At the end of 18 months children can say mama

   c. By 2 years children can utter 2–3 words at a time

   d. At the end of 30 months a child can understand a three-part sentence

   e. It takes 24 hours post-natally for a baby to distinguish its mother's voice

48. Which one of the following is not associated with slow speech development?

   a. Female gender

   b. Prolonged second stage of labour

   c. Large family size

   d. Being one of a twin

   e. Bilingual family

49. The following fears correspond appropriately to the age group, except:

   a. Fear of novel stimuli peaks at 12 months old

   b. Fear of height begins from 6 to 8 months old

   c. Fear of the dark is common in 3- to 5-year-olds

   d. Fear of animals is common in 3- to 5-year-olds

   e. Fear of death is common in adolescence

50. The following are criteria for factitious disorder, except:

   a. Intentional production of physical symptoms

   b. Feigning of psychological symptoms

   c. Behaviour motivated by secondary gain

   d. Avoiding legal responsibility

   e. Munchausen's syndrome

51. Which one of these statements about body dysmorphic disorder is correct?

   a. It starts in early adolescence

   b. It is frequently co-morbid with social phobia

   c. There is a relationship between the degree of deformity and psychological disturbance

   d. It is a form of secondary delusion

   e. Males equal females in prevalence

52. Mr Bond behaves as though limbs on one side of his body are missing during an epileptic aura. This condition is known as:

   a. Hemispatial neglect

   b. Anosognosia

   c. Hemiasomatognosia

   d. Hyperschemazia

   e. Paraschemazia

53. A 29-year-old lady from Cambodia presents with preoccupation of loss of vitality and compulsive wearing of layers of clothes. This condition is known as:

   a. Koro

   b. Frigophobia

   c. Latah

   d. Evil eye

   e. Windigo

54. James starts to realise that he is a boy and that it is different to being a girl. How old is James?

   a. 12 months

   b. 9 months

   c. 15 months

   d. 18 months

   e. 24 months

55. Which one of these statements about neurotransmitters is correct?

   a. For each neuron the same transmitter is released at all its synapses

   b. A neurotransmitter need not always be present at the nerve terminal where it is thought to act

   c. A neurotransmitter is usually released from the nerve terminal following nerve stimulation

   d. A neurotransmitter may activate a postsynaptic receptor site following its release

   e. Enzymes concerned in the synthesis of neurotransmitters should be present in the postsynaptic neuron

56. Which one of these statements about the depolarisation process is correct?

a. Depolarisation closes the sodium channels

b. The falling phase of action potential is caused by closing of the potassium channels

c. In some nerve cells, action potentials are followed by hyperpolarisation

d. It is impossible to trigger an action potential in the refractory period

e. Excitatory neurotransmitters produce excitatory postsynaptic potentials lasting for five seconds

57. Which one of these statements about dopamine receptors is correct?

a. Dopamine is stimulatory on D2 and inhibitory on D1 receptors

b. D2 receptors are positively linked with adenylate cyclase

c. D2 receptors are approximately 15 times more sensitive to the action of dopamine than D1 receptors

d. D2 receptors are located presynaptically on corticostriatal neurons and postsynaptically in the striatum and substantia nigra

e. D4 receptor is of higher density in the cerebellum compared to other brain regions

58. Which one of these statements about 5-HT receptors is correct?

a. Tetrodotoxin blocks potassium and sodium channels leading to paralysis

b. 5-HT-2 receptors are concentrated in the olfactory cortex

c. Ondansetron is a specific 5-HT-1 antagonist

d. Ritanserin is an antagonist of 5-HT-1 and 5-HT-2

e. 5-HT-2 receptors mediate inhibitory impulses in the cortex

59. Which one of these statements is true?

   a. Acetylcholine is inhibitory on M1 and excitatory on M2 receptors

   b. Adrenaline is distributed mainly in fore and midbrain

   c. Presynaptic inhibition occurs in adrenergic, dopaminergic and GABA-ergic synapses

   d. Flumazenil blocks activity of GABA agonist on the GABA-B receptor

   e. Glycerine acts on NMDA receptors

60. Which one of these statements about pharmacokinetics is correct?

   a. In first order kinetics, the rate of elimination of a drug depends directly on the amount of drug present in the body

   b. First order kinetics are followed by drugs when other mechanisms are saturated

   c. Bioequivalence refers to the amount of a drug that has been absorbed

   d. Therapeutic index is the ratio of minimum effective concentration to minimum tolerated concentration

   e. Drugs with large distribution volumes will invariably cross the blood-brain barrier

61. A 69-year-old man admitted to a forensic unit has recently been on a mood stabiliser. He is noted to have disorientation and his MMSE score is below the normal cut-off. His blood test shows altered liver enzymes and hyperammonaemia. Which of these mood stabilisers is he likely to be taking?

   a. Lithium

   b. Olanzapine

   c. Sodium valproate

   d. Carbamazepine

   e. Lamotrigine

62. Which one of the following effects is caused by ECT?

   a. Increased 5-HT-1 receptors

   b. Decreased 5-HT-2 receptors

   c. Increased 5-HT-1 and decreased 5-HT-2

   d. Increased 5-HT-2 only

   e. Decreased 5-HT-1 and increased 5-HT-2

63. A 29-year-old man complains of a headache since being started on a drug that acts on 5-HT-1A receptors. Which of the following drugs is it?

   a. Buspirone

   b. Bupropion

   c. Paraldehyde

   d. Ritanserin

   e. Ondansetron

64. A 63-year-old man complains of halitosis caused by his medication. Which of these drugs is he likely to be taking?

   a. Zaleplon

   b. Zopiclone

   c. Zolpidem

   d. Paraldehyde

   e. Chlordiazepoxide

65. A 42-year-old man has been on antipsychotics for the treatment of catatonic schizophrenia. His EEG would show:

   a. Decreased alpha and theta waves only

   b. Decreased alpha waves and increased theta and delta waves

   c. Decreased delta and increased alpha and theta waves

   d. Increased alpha, theta and delta waves

   e. Decreased alpha, theta and delta waves

66. Mr Rutherford is worried about discontinuation syndrome on SSRIs. You assure him that the risk is minimal with the SSRI he is taking. Which SSRI is it likely to be?

a. Paroxetine

b. Citalopram

c. Sertraline

d. Fluoxetine

e. Escitalopram

67. Mrs Lewis has a long history of depressive episodes with psychotic symptoms and she is on an MAOI. During an inpatient episode, she developed EPSEs and was started on an anticholinergic drug. Since then her physical state has deteriorated and she has become acutely confused. The anticholinergic medication is likely to be:

a. Procyclidine

b. Orphenadrine

c. Tetrabenazine

d. Hyoscine

e. Benzhexol

68. Andrew had a history of refractory seizures and was started on an antiepileptic. Following this he presented to A&E in a psychotic state. On neurological assessment, the FY2 doctor in A&E has found that Andrew has reduced peripheral vision. This could be due to:

a. Gabapentin

b. Vigabatrin

c. Lamotrigine

d. Topiramate

e. Levetiracetam

69. Lithium acts by:

   a. Increasing cAMP production and increasing 5-HT release

   b. Inhibiting phosphoinositide second messenger system

   c. Increasing phosphoinositide second messenger system

   d. Decreasing cAMP production

   e. Inhibiting calcium release

70. A 64-year-old lady has a long history of bipolar affective disorder and is on lithium. She has recently developed symptoms of arthritis and her GP starts her on treatment for this. She develops nausea, coarse tremor and slurred speech. Which of these is likely to have caused the adverse interaction?

   a. Paracetamol

   b. Co-codamol

   c. Ibuprofen

   d. Prednisolone

   e. All the above

71. Which one of these statements about dopamine is correct?

   a. D2 receptors decrease cAMP

   b. Decrease in D2 receptors in brain autopsy confirms schizophrenia

   c. Impairments in cognitive functioning occur in patients but not volunteers after treatment with neuroleptics

   d. Dopaminergic activity of neuroleptics causes primary amenorrhoea

   e. Lens opacities are caused by a dose-related action on D2 receptors

72. Mr Kendall is on a phenothiazine. This will potentiate the effects of all except which one of the following?

   a. Antihistamines

   b. Opioid analgesics

   c. Alcohol

d. Benzodiazepines

e. Lithium

73. Mr Morton, a 69-year-old gentleman, has developed pigmentary retinopathy attributable to his medication. Which of these drugs is he probably taking?

a. Haloperidol

b. Chlorpromazine

c. Trifluoperazine

d. Thioridazine

e. Zuclopenthixol

74. Which one of the following will not increase plasma levels of other drugs?

a. Sodium valproate

b. Cimetidine

c. Imipramine

d. Carbamazepine

e. Metronidazole

75. Mr Johnson has a relapse of psoriasis when started on a mood stabiliser. Which of these drugs has he probably been given?

a. Carbamazepine

b. Lithium

c. Lamotrigine

d. Sodium valproate

e. Olanzapine

76. The therapeutic range of carbamazepine is:

a. 0.8–1.0 mmol/L

b. 1.0–10 mmol/L

c. 20–50 mmol/L

d. 60–80 mmol/L

e. 10–80 mmol/L

77. Which benzodiazepine is rapidly conjugated to an inactive product?

a. Diazepam

b. Lorazepam

c. Oxazepam

d. Nitrazepam

e. Chlordiazepoxide

78. Which phase in a clinical trial is aimed at establishing the incidence of side-effects in a patient population?

a. Phase 1a

b. Phase 1b

c. Phase 2

d. Phase 3

e. Phase 4

79. Mr Richards has developed tremor from being on lithium. (The lithium level is in therapeutic range.) Tremor can be treated with:

a. Propranolol

b. Procyclidine

c. Tetrabenazine

d. Diazepam

e. Benzhexol

80. Which one of these drugs is a partial agonist of GABA receptors?

a. Pregabalin

b. Flumazenil

c. Clonazepam

d. Diazepam

e. Beta-CCE

81. Martin, an OT staff member in a psychiatric unit, had been diagnosed with seasonal affective disorder. Which of the following is not true about his illness?

    a. Morning treatment with light therapy is better

    b. Light therapy dosage is 2500 lux, 2 hours a day

    c. There is a one in two chance that his brother might have depression

    d. His illness, left untreated, would probably resolve by spring time

    e. He would crave for carbohydrate foods

82. Mrs Stevens would like to know about factors that affect the chances of her recovery from bipolar affective disorder. Which among the following statements is correct?

    a. The likelihood of a switch to bipolar disorder increases after the third episode of depression

    b. The mean age of hospitalisation of someone with bipolar affective disorder is 26 years

    c. Agitation is a factor that could have predicted a switch from depression to bipolar affective disorder

    d. Her high score on neuroticism dimension on EPI is associated with faster recovery

    e. Hallucinations predict a faster recovery

83. Mr Parker is on treatment with lithium for bipolar affective disorder. Which one of these statements is true?

    a. As his parents and two of his brothers suffer from the same illness, he has a poorer chance of a good prognosis on lithium

    b. Recent studies have indicated that the serum lithium level needed for prophylaxis is lower than was thought when he commenced it 10 years ago

    c. Twitching is a sign of mild lithium toxicity when he is taking ibuprofen along with lithium

    d. The chance of him going bald on lithium is 1%

    e. His brother, in rapid cycling phase, will benefit from lithium

84. Mr Simpson is worried about the risk of bipolar affective disorder after having watched Stephen Fry's TV programme on the subject. Which of the following statements is true about the risk of bipolar disorder?

    a. In men, dysthymia is more common than bipolar affective disorder

    b. Had he developed unipolar depression and belonged to a Bangladeshi background, his risk of depression would have been higher than his sister

    c. As he has always been single, his risk of depression is low

    d. As his brother has depression, the risk of Mr Simpson developing bipolar affective disorder is greater than that of the general population

    e. Low 5-HIAA level in the CSF is a marker for depression

85. Mrs Hilda Smith is a 73-year-old lady on amitriptyline. Which of the following is true?

    a. A steady-state concentration of drug would have been achieved in 3 days

    b. Amitriptyline is safer than lofepramine in overdose

    c. Amitriptyline causes mydriasis

    d. Amitriptyline causes increased T-wave amplitude on ECG

    e. Hypernatraemia is a common feature

86. Mrs Benedict is treated with an SSRI. Which of these statements is not true about SSRI treatment?

    a. A minimum of 2 weeks should be allowed before changing over to an SSRI from phenelzine

    b. Citalopram is a weak inhibitor of CYP450

    c. 75% of orally administered fluoxetine reaches the systemic circulation

    d. Cimetidine delays the excretion of citalopram

    e. Diaphoresis can possibly indicate serotonin syndrome

87. Which one of these statements about ECT is correct?

    a. Premorbid personality factors predict a good response to ECT

b. ECT is less effective in schizophrenic patients presenting with delusions of passivity

c. Old age reduces the seizure threshold

d. Females have a lower seizure threshold

e. Hypoxia prolongs the duration of seizure in ECT

88. Which one of these statements about psychotherapy for depression is correct?

a. Cognitive therapy uses a graded task assignment

b. Reality testing is a behaviour technique used in cognitive therapy

c. Interpersonal psychotherapy (IPT) lasts for 3–4 months

d. The marital relationship is the focus of IPT

e. Childhood experiences are crucial to IPT

89. Which of the following associations is true with regard to measuring cognitive impairment in schizophrenia?

a. Wisconsin Card Sorting Test – attention and concentration

b. Stroop test – executive functioning

c. Continuous Performance Test – selective attention

d. Word generation task – executive functioning

e. NART – IQ following the onset of illness

90. Which one of these statements about schizophrenia is correct?

a. A family history of bipolar affective disorder in Mr Robinson's dad is a good prognostic sign

b. According to ICD-10 the prodromal non-psychotic phase should be included in the duration criteria

c. Afro-Caribbean immigrants have a higher risk of schizophrenia in the UK, but not in their country of origin

d. The temporal horn of the left ventricle is reduced in schizophrenia

e. In the Camberwell family interview, scorings are based on content

91. Mr Smith has been diagnosed with vascular dementia. Pathological features of this condition include all, except:

a. Microscopic infarcts

b. Macroscopic infarcts

c. Ventricular dilatation

d. Selective asymmetrical atrophy of the temporal lobes

e. Generalised cerebral atrophy

92. Excessive eating occurs in:

a. Prader-Willi Syndrome

b. Angelman's syndrome

c. William's syndrome

d. Klinefelter's syndrome

e. Munchausen's syndrome

93. Mr Cooper has presented homeless and in a poor nutritional state. His cyanocobalamin level is low. Which one of the following is a likely mental health complication?

a. Depression

b. Delirium

c. Reversible dementia

d. Paranoia

e. Anxiety

94. Mr Jones has a stroke involving the non-dominant temporal lobe. The following are possible neurological deficits, except:

a. Hemiasomatognosia

b. Prosopagnosia

c. Amusia

d. Impaired ability to reproduce visual designs from memory

e. Epilepsy

95. Joan has been diagnosed with anorexia nervosa. Which of the following is not a likely symptom:

a. Loss of at least 25% of body weight

b. Loss of pubic hair

c. Episodes of self-harm

d. Amenorrhoea before significant weight loss

e. Loss of libido

96. Which one of these statements about head injury is correct?

a. Persisting cognitive impairment occurs when there is post-traumatic amnesia between 1 and 12 hours

b. It is more common in the young

c. Recovery stops at 6 months

d. It has no association with amount of brain damage

e. It more commonly damages the dominant hemisphere

97. A 29-year-old Afro Caribbean male had elevated CPK following an increase of his antipsychotic medication. The following symptoms would have been suggestive of neuroleptic malignant syndrome (NMS), except:

a. Autonomic dysfunction

b. Mutism

c. Rigidity

d. Diaphoresis

e. Hyperthermia

98. Mr Romsey had recently lost his wife from cancer. The following are symptoms of normal grief reaction, except:

a. Sadness

b. Weeping

c. Poor concentration

d. Impaired memory

e. Guilt

99. Mr Denver experienced a huge loss of money due to investing in hedge funds. Within half an hour of his company collapsing he wandered off and didn't return home for two days. What is this behaviour called?

    a. Hysterical fugue

    b. Organic fugue state

    c. Adjustment disorder

    d. Acute stress reaction

    e. Post-traumatic stress disorder (PTSD)

100. Differential diagnosis of depersonalisation includes all, except:

    a. Depression

    b. Schizophrenia

    c. Mania

    d. Dissociative disorder

    e. Temporal lobe epilepsy

101. Which one of these statements about rTMS is correct?

    a. It stimulates the sub-cortical areas

    b. The magnetic field penetrates the cortex to a depth of 1 cm

    c. A coil situated at the vertex stimulates the small muscles of the hand

    d. The time for stimulation remains static during a course of treatment

    e. In schizophrenia it particularly reduces paranoia

102. Which one of these drugs is an antipsychotic that has an active metabolite?

    a. Olanzapine

    b. Risperidone

    c. Quetiapine

    d. Aripiprazole

    e. Sertindole

103. Mr Kendal is started on an anticholinergic drug for EPSE. He then starts to experience insomnia. Which of these drugs is most likely to cause this?

    a. Benzhexol

    b. Benztropine

    c. Biperiden

    d. Orphenadrine

    e. Procyclidine

104. Mr Foyle is not on antipsychotic medication, but complains of restless legs. This would respond best to:

    a. Orphenadrine

    b. L-Dopa

    c. Cyproheptadine

    d. Propranolol

    e. Diazepam

105. Mr Wallace has a history of 'dry sex' without impairment of libido, orgasm or erection, while taking one of these antipsychotics. Which one is it likely to be?

    a. Risperidone

    b. Olanzapine

    c. Sertindole

    d. Ziprasidone

    e. Quetiapine

106. Oculodermal melanosis is a side effect of which one of these antipsychotics?

    a. Thienobenzodiazepine

    b. Dibenzodiazepine

    c. Benzamide

    d. Benzisoxazole

    e. Phenothiazines

107. Clinical hepatitis has been reported with which one of these medications?

    a. Risperidone

    b. Olanzapine

    c. Quetiapine

    d. Amisulpride

    e. Aripiprazole

108. A child has developed absence seizures. The first line drug would be:

    a. Lamotrigine

    b. Gabapentin

    c. Levetiracetam

    d. Topiramate

    e. Vigabatrin

109. The drug with the least protein binding is:

    a. Sodium valproate

    b. Carbamazepine

    c. Lamotrigine

    d. Phenytoin

    e. Ethosuximide

110. Mr Summers reports loss of visual field since starting on an antiepileptic. Which one of these is it likely to be?

    a. Gabapentin

    b. Tiagabine

    c. Vigabatrin

    d. Levetiracetam

    e. Lamotrigine

111. Which one of the following age-related pharmacokinetic mechanisms is not true in the elderly?

    a. Increased receptor sensitivity

    b. Decreased plasma albumin

c. Decreased blood-levels of water soluble drugs

d. Decreased GFR

e. Prolonged half-life of lipid soluble drugs

112. Side-effects from SSRIs due to their activity on 5-HT-2 receptors include all the following, except:

a. Agitation

b. Akathisia

c. Weight gain

d. Insomnia

e. Sexual dysfunction

113. Mr Peterson develops a headache since starting treatment for Alzheimer's dementia. Which of following medications is likely to be the cause?

a. Galantamine

b. Rivastigmine

c. Donepezil

d. All of the above

e. None of the above

114. Which one of these statements about the DSM-IV and ICD-10 is correct?

a. DSM–IV requires two out of three essential symptoms

b. There is a higher threshold for 'mild' depressive episodes in ICD-10

c. Partial remission according to DSM-IV requires no signs or symptoms during the last 2 months

d. In ICD-10, psychotic symptoms include depressive stupor

e. According to DSM-IV, delusion of persecution is mood congruent

115. A 49-year-old lady presents with monthly depressive episodes that last for less than 2 weeks, and is relatively free of depression otherwise. What is the name of this condition?

    a. Recurrent depressive disorder

    b. Cyclothymia

    c. Dysthymia

    d. Double depression

    e. Brief recurrent depressive disorder

116. Which one of these statements about rating scales for depression is correct?

    a. Beck's Depression Inventory has 17 items

    b. MADRS has 10 items and requires a clinical interview

    c. Zung Self-Rating Depression Scale has an imbalance towards the psychological phenomena

    d. Wakefield Self-Assessment Inventory includes an anxiety scale

    e. An advantage of the visual analogue scale is that it avoids contrast effects.

117. The following are types of mania according to Kraepelin, except for:

    a. Hypomania

    b. Delirious mania

    c. Chronic mania

    d. Dysphoric mania

    e. Acute mania

118. Which one of the following was described by Kahlbaum?

    a. Dysthymia

    b. Cyclothymia

    c. Reactive depression

    d. Hypomania

    e. Double depression

119. Unipolar depressives with a family history of mania are sometimes known as:

a. BP-III

b. BP-IV

c. md

d. MD

e. Pseudo-bipolar

120. Which one of these statements about rapid cycling is not true?

a. Rapid cycling has been described in secondary mania associated with organic brain disease

b. Some cases are associated with clinical hypothyroidism

c. Some cases are associated with sub-clinical hypothyroidism

d. Ultra rapid cycling is the term used when mood changes oscillate every 48 hours

e. Rapid cycling is defined as having three or more affective episodes every year

121. Secondary mania is associated with the addition of the following medications, except:

a. Bromocriptine

b. Clonidine

c. Levothyroxine

d. Procyclidine

e. Amphetamine

122. Signs of mild lithium toxicity include all, except:

a. Nausea

b. Vomiting

c. Diarrhoea

d. Severe fine tremor

e. Poor concentration

123. Which one of these statements about the neuroendocrine hypothesis of depression is not correct?

    a. A small proportion of patients show an exaggerated TSH response to hypothalamic TRH

    b. Elevated cortisol secretion and non-DST suppression relate to poor prognosis, but not cognitive failure

    c. PRL response to 5-HT agonists is reduced in depression

    d. GH response to alpha-2 adrenoceptor agonists is reduced

    e. In unipolar depression and seasonal affective disorder, melatonin levels and rhythms are normal

124. Factors that increase the risk of prison suicide include all, except:

    a. Age < 30 years

    b. Being in remand

    c. A long sentence

    d. Previous deliberate self-harm (DSH)

    e. Conviction for a serious offence

125. Factors that increase the risk of suicide in alcohol addicts include all, except:

    a. Being male

    b. Peak age 40–60 years

    c. Poor work record in the last 5 years

    d. Social isolation

    e. Previous DSH

126. With regard to suicide prevention which one of these statements is correct?

    a. Removal of toxic coal-gas reduced suicide by 50%

    b. 68% of people over the age of 65 who committed suicide had seen their GP in the four weeks before death

    c. There is some evidence that elderly white women benefit from speaking to the Samaritans

d. Substance misuse in young people without a previous history of DSH is specifically associated with suicide

e. Suicide rates are higher in spring in the northern hemisphere and winter in the southern hemisphere

127. With regard to deliberate self-harm which one of these statements is correct?

a. In the month following a life event, the risk of DSH is 10 times that of the general population

b. Being in debt is the single most common event reported for DSH

c. There is a higher level of 5-HIAA in those with a history of DSH compared to those without a history of DSH

d. Hopelessness is associated with suicide, but not with DSH

e. DSH is less common in people younger than 25 years

128. Risk factors for suicide in patients admitted to hospital following DSH include:

a. Being female

b. Older age in men and women

c. Repeated attempts of DSH

d. Short-term use of hypnotics

e. Good physical health

129. After being sacked at work, Mr Johnson presents in a dazed state with narrowed attention and disorientation, and he becomes overactive in A&E. Examination reveals tachycardia, sweating and flushing. What is his condition called?

a. Panic disorder without agoraphobia

b. PTSD

c. Generalised anxiety disorder (GAD)

d. Adjustment disorder

e. Acute stress reaction

130. DSM criteria for adjustment disorder include all, except:
    a. Emotional symptoms occurring within 6 months of an identifiable stressor
    b. Symptoms lasting than 3 months once the stressor is terminated
    c. Detachment or estrangement from others
    d. Distress not greater than expected from exposure to the stressor
    e. Symptoms not due to bereavement

131. Specific symptoms of benzodiazepine withdrawal syndrome include all, except:
    a. Photophobia
    b. Tinnitus
    c. Tremor
    d. Muscle twitching
    e. Hyper-reflexia

132. With regard to phobias which one of these statements is correct?
    a. Agoraphobia is associated with urgency of micturition
    b. Fear of seeing friends or acquaintances is seen in social phobia
    c. Relatives of patients with agoraphobia are at increased risk of agoraphobia and other phobias
    d. Social phobia is commonest among phobias
    e. Agoraphobia shows a peak at the age of 35

133. The following are categories of somatoform disorder in the ICD-10, except:
    a. Undifferentiated somatoform disorder
    b. Persistent pain disorder
    c. Neurasthenia
    d. Body dysmorphic disorder
    e. Other somatoform disorders

134. Which one of the following is a predictor of good outcome in conversion disorder?

  a. Long history

  b. Young age

  c. Personality disorder

  d. Disability benefit

  e. Involvement in litigation

135. With regard to secondary sleep disorders which one of these statements is correct?

  a. Focal frontal lobe seizures occur commonly during NREM sleep

  b. Fibromyalgia shows characteristic alpha wave intrusion into sleep EEG

  c. Acute amphetamine withdrawal is associated with increased REM and reduced stage 3 and 4

  d. Rebound phenomena following benzodiazepine discontinuation are associated with decreased REM

  e. SSRIs decrease sleep fragmentation

Paper 4

4

1. 'Motor scheme' was coined by:
   a. Beck
   b. Sullivan
   c. Freud
   d. Roger
   e. Piaget

2. The rattle experiment, using a child wired for physiological monitoring, was performed by:
   a. Piaget in sensorimotor stage in a 3-month-old child
   b. Bower in sensorimotor stage to establish physiological evidence for difficulty in conceiving objects
   c. Bower in a 24-month-old child to prove Piaget's theory
   d. Piaget in a 24-month-old child
   e. Bower in a 3-month-old child in sensorimotor stage

3. Social learning theory is associated with all, except:
   a. Bandura
   b. Keehn
   c. Yando
   d. Hayden
   e. Schloss

4. The cocktail party effect is associated with:
   a. Experiments on sustained attention
   b. Shadowing task to test visual attention
   c. Focussed attention
   d. Establishing dual-task interference
   e. Flexibility of divided attention is not a good predictor

5. At which of stage of child development does the game of peek-a-boo usually become evident?
   a. Sensorimotor
   b. Preoperational
   c. Formal operations
   d. Concrete operations
   e. Informal operations

6. A Psychiatry trainee, who believes that he is an excellent psychiatrist, has failed Membership a dozen times. He believes that the exam is non-clinical, ridiculously factual and not a fair indicator of a good clinician. The psychological process applied is:
   a. Cognitive dissonance
   b. Attitude-discrepant behaviour
   c. Hierarchy of needs
   d. Need for achievement
   e. None of the above

7. Which one of these statements is true?
   a. The maxim of relevance is the most important of conversational maxims
   b. The literal meaning of what we say conveys illocutionary force
   c. In a garden path sentence, the human sentence parser is correctly led on hearing the first few words
   d. Lexicon is a pragmatic mental construct resembling a dictionary
   e. According to Vygotsky, linguistic and cognitive development

interact with each other in early childhood to develop internal speech

8. Which one of these statements is true?
   a. Sapir-Whorf hypothesised that thought determines language
   a. The abovementioned principle is linguistic relativism
   b. The dual code theory states that different types of information, though representationally distinct, are processed by the same cognitive processing systems
   c. According to the decompositional view, the meanings of words consist of a number of semantic features
   d. Prototype involves hierarchical representation of meanings of words

9. Which one of these statements about object permanence is correct?
   a. At 6 months an infant will recognise its care-giver
   b. At 6 months the infant understands that objects still exist even though they may not be visible and therefore does not show distress at the care-giver's departure
   c. At 6 months the attachment figure is conceptualised to be in unity with the infant
   d. Fear response to strangers begins at 8 months
   e. Attachment to other children starts in the second year

10. Which of these statements about bonding and attachment is correct?
    a. A primary attachment figure will be a person who provides the most physical care of a child
    b. Children who have suffered severe deprivation cannot form stable attachments in later life
    c. A critical period for forming attachments is the first 2 years
    d. The ability to interact with 'age mates' has a protective effect against the absence of adult attachment
    e. 'Sensitive responsiveness' is an objective measure of parenting behaviour described by Ainsworth

11. Which one of these statements about 'Strange Situation' is correct?

   a. It is tested in 1 year old infants

   b. It is carried out in the infant's home environment

   c. One-third of the children showed avoidance behaviour

   d. Secure children showed little exploratory behaviour in the absence of a mother

   e. Ambivalent children showed anxiety at reunion

12. Which one of these statements about Ainsworth's findings is correct?

   a. Proximity-seeking behaviour correlates directly with the strength of attachment

   b. A child's behaviour in a strange situation is a function of the mother's temperament

   c. Two-thirds from the 'Strange Situation' belong to the deviant group

   d. In the home situation, there was a difference between mothers

   e. Category A mothers were insensitive

13. Which one of these statements about functions of attachment is correct?

   a. Category A children in peer relationships behave as victims

   b. Category C children behave as victimisers

   c. There is a gender difference in peer-directed social behaviour of insecurely attached children

   d. Bowlby proposed that lack of attachment can be caused by disharmony at home

   e. Dysthymic patients show Category C and D attachment in early childhood

14. A 3-year-old boy has a magic cloth on his head and assumes that since he cannot see others, others cannot see him. He is pleased with this hiding place. What is the term for this way of thinking?

   a. Precausal reasoning

b. Circular reaction

c. Artificialism

d. Propositional thought

e. Egocentricity

15. A 4-year-old boy claims that the wall is hurt when a nail is driven into it. The concept is known as:

a. Schema

b. Animism

c. Artificialism

d. Syncretism

e. Circular reaction

16. A 36-year-old man who sustained a head injury has problems interpreting pictures. When looking at a photograph from his skiing holiday he can say that it contains different colours, but cannot name them. He can point to mountains and people, but cannot say that the photo depicts a group of people skiing. This condition is known as:

a. Agraphaesthesia

b. Reduplicative paramnesia

c. Autotopagnosia

d. Prosopagnosia

e. Simultagnosia

17. A boy believes in obeying rules laid down by the teacher. The boy is at which stage of development?

a. Pre-conventional stage

b. Conventional stage

c. Post-conventional stage

d. Automatic obedience

e. None of the above

18. A 2-year-old boy shows a mug to his brother and says 'Mummy cup.' Which stage of development is this?

a. Prelinguistic stage

b. Critical period

c. Telegraphic period

d. Babbling

e. Transformational grammar

19. Betty, a 19-year-old, claims that she is being stalked by her ex. She points to various men at different tube stations and says that he comes to torment her in different guises, including that of Bruce Forsythe. What is this condition known as?

a. Capgras' syndrome

b. De Clérambault's syndrome

c. Fregoli's syndrome

d. Othello syndrome

e. Delusional erotomania

20. Mrs Bygrave, who is 82, is assessed under Section 3 of the MHA. She has stopped eating and drinking and hardly gets out of her settee. She believes that her stomach and bowels have decayed. What is this condition known as?

a. Charles Bonnet syndrome

b. Cotard's syndrome

c. Ekbom's syndrome

d. Couvade syndrome

e. Briquet's syndrome

21. A mother with a long history of borderline personality disorder brings her 2-year-old boy to the A&E claiming that he had vomited blood. The nurse practitioner is concerned that the mother has brought the child in a number of times with different sets of complaints and that no specific pathology has been found on any occasion. What is this condition known as?

a. Briquet's syndrome

b. Polle's syndrome

c. Factitious disorder

d. Dissociative fugue

e. None of the above

22. Mr and Mrs Hall are expecting their first baby and Mrs Hall is booked for her dating scan. Mr Smith turns up to his GP on the day of the scan claiming sickness, abdominal discomfort and a distended abdomen. On examination he is normal. What is this condition known as?

a. Malingering

b. Factitious disorder

c. Briquet's syndrome

d. Couvade syndrome

e. Adjustment disorder

23. After being hounded in the House of Commons about the Northern Rock, the Chancellor of the Exchequer returned to Number 11 and shouted at his Principal Secretary. The defence mechanism he displayed is known as:

a. Projection

b. Reaction formation

c. Displacement

d. Aggression

e. Conversion

24. A neurologist describes a 69-year-old man in a geriatric unit as being in a twilight state. Which one of these statements is not true of this condition?

a. It occurs in the context of mania a potu

b. It can last up to several weeks

c. It can be used as a legal defence

d. It starts gradually

e. The Ganser state is a sort of twilight state

25. A 27-year-old man has recently been diagnosed with epilepsy and his wife is very concerned about his 'automatisms'. Which one of these statements is not true about automatisms?

   a. Her husband could have an automatism following a seizure with full control of posture and muscle tone

   b. An aura could be a temporal lobe automatism

   c. Behaviour during an automatism is usually inappropriate

   d. Violence is rare during an automatism

   e. During an automatism, her husband would retain an awareness of the environment

26. Which one of these statements is not true?

   a. Occupational delirium could be seen in an oneiroid state

   b. Relational functions are present in stupor

   c. A 72-year-old man with locked-in syndrome has disruptions of the motor pathways to the pons

   d. A person with akinetic mutism would generally have clouding of consciousness

   e. Symptoms of akinetic mutism can occur in a conscious patient with schizophrenia

27. Attention is best defined as:

   a. A subjective description of a state in which percepts may be received

   b. Sustained perception for a period of time

   c. Objective observation of another person or event

   d. The capacity of a person to gauge time, space and person in the current setting

   e. Orientation to time and place

28. Which one of these statements about EEG is correct?

   a. A person in stage 3 sleep will show large amounts of high amplitude and slow wave activity

   b. A person in REM sleep will show relatively low voltage and mixed frequency activity

c. A person in stage 2 sleep will show large amounts of high amplitude and slow wave activity

d. A person in stage 1 sleep will show sleep spindles

e. A person in stage 4 sleep will show low voltage and mixed frequency without eye movement

29. Which one of these concepts is not associated with Donald Winnicott?

a. Pathological mother

b. Object permanence

c. Transitional object

d. Holding environment

e. Potential space

30. According to Erikson, obsessions are found during which of the following psychosocial stages:

a. Generativity vs. stagnation

b. Initiative vs. guilt

c. Industry vs. inferiority

d. Autonomy vs. shame

e. Trust vs. mistrust

31. Jennifer complains of a voice speaking her thoughts aloud exactly at same time that she thinks. This condition is known as:

a. Echo de la pensee

b. Gedankenlautwerden

c. Verbigeration

d. Running commentary

e. Second rank symptoms of schizophrenia

32. A 79-year-old retired reverend is admitted to the EMAU with an altered state of consciousness in which he goes around offering blessing and asking for confessions. What is the name of his condition?

    a. Drowsiness

    b. Twilight state

    c. Oneiroid state

    d. Sopor

    e. Coma

33. Korsakoff's psychosis involves a lesion of the:

    a. Associate motor speech area

    b. Hypothalamic nucleus

    c. Putamen

    d. Mamillary body

    e. Subthalamic nucleus

34. Which of these is not a false perception?

    a. Pareidolia

    b. Splitting

    c. Illusions

    d. Hallucinations

    e. Pseudohallucinations

35. In a delirious episode, Mr Stewart claims to see '. . . a Victorian lady with a crinoline and frilled bloomers . . .'. What is the name of his condition?

    a. Completion illusion

    b. Affect illusion

    c. Pareidolia

    d. Perceptual misinterpretation

    e. Fantastic interpretation

36. 'The curtains were moved and I knew that my nephew had written a book about me depicting me as a pervert.' What is the name of this condition?
    a. Reflex hallucination
    b. Functional hallucination
    c. Delusional perception
    d. Extracampine hallucination
    e. Nihilistic delusion

37. Which one of these is not associated with Charles Bonnet syndrome?
    a. Central reduction in vision
    b. Peripheral reduction in vision
    c. Phantom visual image
    d. Absence of demonstrable psychopathology
    e. Dementia

38. Reverse autoscopy is commonly associated with:
    a. Generalised anxiety disorder
    b. Dementia
    c. Depression
    d. Paranoid schizophrenia
    e. Social phobia

39. The term 'Cognitive Dissonance' was coined by:
    a. McClelland
    b. Beck
    c. Festinger
    d. Bard
    e. Schachter

40. Cognitive dissonance:

   a. Reduces internal discomfort

   b. Is associated with decreased arousal

   c. Is associated with situations when cognition and behaviour are inconsistent

   d. Does not lead to change in individual's behaviour

41. Which one of these statements about operant conditioning is correct?

   a. It is one form of associative learning

   b. It cannot be used in patients with dementia and learning disability

   c. It is successful with punishment

   d. Negative reinforcement refers to the reinforcement of a response through the addition of a negative reinforcer

   e. All of the above

42. Which one of the following is not a type of social power?

   a. Cohesive

   b. Expert

   c. Authoritative

   d. Coercive

   e. Referent

43. Which one of these statements about types of thinking is correct?

   a. According to Fish, there are four types of thinking

   b. Undirected fantasy thinking is also called dereistic thinking

   c. Functions of thinking are manifest in a phenomenon

   d. De Bono is associated with thinking in shy, mentally-well people

   e. Maternal reverie is a form of autistic thinking

44. Which one of these statements about flight of ideas is not true?

   a. The goal of thinking is not maintained for long

b. Acceleration of flow of thinking occurs

c. Determining tendency is weakened

d. Loosening of association is present

e. There is logical connection between two expressed ideas

45. 'They said I was in the pantry at home . . . Peekaboo . . . there's a magic box. Poor darling Catherine, you know, Catherine the Great, the fire grate, I'm always up the chimney.' Thinking and speaking in this way is known as:

a. Circumstantiality

b. Loosening of association

c. Flight of ideas

d. Verbigeration

e. Derailment

46. Which one of these paired associations is not true?

a. Circumstantial thinking – failure of differentiation of figure ground

b. Verschmelzung – fusion

c. Faseln – muddling

d. Judgement – thought that expresses reality

e. Snapping off – thought block

47. 'Traffic is rumbling along the main road. They are going north. Why do girls always play panto heroes?' Thinking and speaking in this way is known as:

a. Muddling

b. Derailment

c. Fusion

d. Snapping off

e. Crowding

48. I know that I am biologically a man, but it is a horrible freak of nature. Really I am a woman and by some accident I have a male body.' A statement of this nature is characteristic of:

    a. Transsexualism

    b. Transvestism

    c. Egodystonic sexual orientation

    d. Couvade syndrome

    e. Turner's syndrome

49. Which one of these statements is not true?

    a. Psychogenic pain is sporadic

    b. Psychogenic pain is diffuse

    c. Facial pain is associated with obsessive personality

    d. Abdominal pain in childhood relates to hypochondriacal disorder in adult life

    e. Vital feelings is the localisation of depression in a bodily organ

50. Affect is:

    a. Positive or negative reaction to an experience

    b. Differentiated specific feelings directed towards objects

    c. Prevailing disposition

    d. Physiological or psychological concomitant of mood

    e. Subjective evaluation of mood

51. Lack of emotional sensitivity in 69-year-old Mr O'Grady is:

    a. Apathy

    b. Flattening

    c. Blunting

    d. Anhedonia

    e. Alexithymia

52. 'Flowers open for me.' This thought could be associated with:

    a. Anhedonia

    b. Elation

    c. Euphoria

d. Ecstasy

e. Lability

53. Mr Lampard complains of having sensations of being strangled. What is this condition?

a. Kinaesthetic hallucination

b. Visceral hallucination

c. Haptic hallucination

d. Hygric hallucination

e. Somatic passivity

54. Mr Kumar has been diagnosed with pseudobulbar palsy. Which one of these features is not consistent with this diagnosis?

a. Dysarthria

b. Dysphagia

c. Absent jaw jerk

d. Fasciculation of facial muscles

e. Wasting of the tongue

55. Important features of supportive psychotherapy include all, except:

a. Listening

b. Explanation

c. Prestige suggestion

d. Reassurance

e. Countertransference

56. According to Freud:

a. Id functions by secondary process thinking

b. Id obeys the reality principle

c. Transference is analysed

d. The conscious, subconscious and preconscious form a structural model of the mind

e. The phallic phase is the last phase in psychosexual development

57. Which one of the following is a mature defence mechanism?

   a. Rationalisation

   b. Reaction formation

   c. Undoing

   d. Sublimation

   e. Displacement

58. Which one of these conditions is considered to be a dissociative disorder?

   a. Somatisation

   b. Somatoform autonomic dysfunction

   c. Hypochondriasis

   d. Ganser's syndrome

   e. Factitious disorder

59. David, a 27-year-old single unemployed male, presents with fear of blushing. Which one of the following conditions is he suffering from?

   a. Agoraphobia

   b. Panic disorder with agoraphobia

   c. Social phobia

   d. Generalised anxiety disorder

   e. Hebephrenic schizophrenia

60. A 27-year-old lady with post partum depression is admitted to the mother and baby unit. She is found to be agitated at night and the nurse rings you for a benzodiazepine. Which one should be prescribed?

   a. Chlordiazepoxide

   b. Zopiclone

   c. Lorazepam

   d. Diazepam

   e. Temazepam

61. The obstetric and gynaecology registrar mentions to you that a mother is on a particular antidepressant. In your opinion, it does not cause side-effects to a breast-feeding infant. Which antidepressant is it?

a. Amitriptyline

b. Dothiepin

c. Clomipramine

d. Venlafaxine

e. Mirtazapine

62. A 49-year-old lady gains weight after starting on an antidepressant for depression with biological symptoms. Which antidepressant is it likely to be?

a. Venlafaxine

b. Nefazadone

c. Mirtazapine

d. Reboxetine

e. Amitriptyline

63. Mr Wilson has been on clozapine for 3 weeks when he attends the Clozaril clinic. The nurse practitioner is concerned that his temperature is 38.7 degrees. What would you do?

a. Admit the patient to the hospital

b. Refer the patient to a cardiologist

c. Reduce the dose of clozapine

d. Arrange for FBC

e. All of the above

64. A 36-year-old lady with COPD is started on an antidepressant. After taking some cough mixture she develops sweating, nausea and headache. What antidepressant is she on?

a. Phenelzine

b. Reboxetine

c. Venlafaxine

d. Nortriptyline

e. Pimozide

65. Which one of the following is not a side-effect of reboxetine?

a. Insomnia

b. Dry mouth

c. Constipation

d. Weight gain

e. All of the above

66. A 49-year-old man who is taking an antipsychotic following a relapse of schizophrenia, feels exhausted when he wakes and has missed OT sessions. He has gained 9 kg in weight and has been started on lactulose. Which antipsychotic is he on?

a. Quetiapine

b. Risperidone

c. Amisulpride

d. Aripiprazole

e. Clozapine

67. Mr Schmidt has been on lithium as an augmentation for treating depression. He has recently been started on bendroflumethiazide. Which of the following is not a sign of lithium toxicity?

a. Coarse tremor

b. Disorientation

c. Polydipsia

d. Slurred speech

e. Vomiting

68. Mrs Benmar develops an episode of seizure following initiation of an antidepressant medication. Which one of these drugs has she probably been given?

a. Fluvoxamine

b. Mianserin

c. Maprotiline

d. Phenelzine

e. Tranylcypromine

69. Which one of these statements about GABA receptors is not correct?

    a. GABA is inhibitory
    b. GABA-A is linked to a postsynaptic chloride channel
    c. Benzodiazepines bind to benzodiazepine receptors and not GABA receptors
    d. GABA-A mediates the activity of benzodiazepine
    e. GABA-B mediates the activity of barbiturates

70. Mrs Waller has developed DVT and is to be commenced on warfarin. Her physician is concerned about her taking which of the following antidepressant medications?

    a. Imipramine
    b. Venlafaxine
    c. Mirtazapine
    d. Fluoxetine
    e. Trazodone

71. Mrs Hollins has recommenced an antidepressant that had benefited her during her first depressive episode 8 years ago. She had been on Epilim Chrono for a long time. You are called as she has had a fit. Which antidepressant could have caused it?

    a. Amitriptyline
    b. Mirtazapine
    c. Trazodone
    d. Nefazadone
    e. Citalopram

72. Mr Hockridge developed acute dystonia after being given a tablet to deal with his GI symptoms, and you discover that he has been taking haloperidol for years as a treatment for motor tics. The tablet given was probably:

    a. Ondansetron
    b. Ranitidine
    c. Omeprazole
    d. Metoclopramide
    e. Senna

73. Mr Hastings, who is on lithium treatment for resistant depression, develops neurotoxicity when started on another drug by the cardiologists. Which one of these is likely to be responsible?
    a. Amiodarone
    b. Aspirin
    c. Verapamil
    d. Digoxin
    e. Perindopril

74. Haloperidol was synthesised by:
    a. Kane
    b. Sternbach
    c. Janssen
    d. Cade
    e. Delay and Deniker

75. With regard to the half-life of drugs (in hours), which one of the following pairings is correct?
    a. Temazepam: 20
    b. Zopiclone: 3–4
    c. Lorazepam: 6–8
    d. Zolpidem: 4–6
    e. Alprazolam: 1–5

76. Which one of the following is true with regard to total sleep time?
    a. Stage 1 – 8%
    b. Stage 2 – 5%
    c. Stage 3 – 12%
    d. Stage 4 – 50%
    e. REM – 25%

77. Tolerance occurs with:

   a. Zopiclone

   b. Zolpidem

   c. Zaleplon

   d. All the above

   e. None of the above

78. Which one of these SSRIs is licensed for use in males and females with PTSD?

   a. Sertraline

   b. Paroxetine

   c. Fluoxetine

   d. Fluvoxamine

   e. Citalopram

79. Mrs Paget, a 32-year-old-cleaner, had multiple episodes of depression in a year. Each episode was moderate in severity and lasted for about 4 days. The diagnosis is:

   a. Dysthymia

   b. Cyclothymia

   c. Brief recurrent depressive disorder

   d. Depression NOS

   e. Acute stress reactions

80. Following the suicide death of a patient in your ward, you are invited by the coroner to answer a few questions about suicide and self-harm. Which one of these statements is true?

   a. A regressing linear curve is obtained when suicide across all social classes is plotted

   b. Social class 5 is associated with deliberate self-harm

   c. Males under 23 years are associated with DSH

   d. Recent use of hypnotics increases risk of suicide

   e. Repeated self-harm is not a risk factor for suicide

81. Harry suffers from PTSD following his stint in Afghanistan. Which one of these statements about PTSD is true?
    a. The Impact of Events Scale has two sub-scales with 15 items each
    b. According to ICD-10, the onset of illness should be 10 months after a traumatic event
    c. Debriefing plays a very important role in treatment
    d. Ganser's syndrome is one variant of PTSD
    e. Intrusive memories tend to be of shorter duration

82. Which one of the following statements is not true?
    a. According to ICD-10, hypochondriacal disorder does not respond to medical reassurance
    b. The Whitley index is a measure of hysteria
    c. Dysmorphophobia is not associated with generalised disturbance of body image
    d. Resistance to thought is always present in dysmorphophobia,
    e. 5% of perpetrators of Munchausen's by proxy are fathers

83. Which one of these statements about personality disorders is not true?
    a. Antisocial personality disorder is a category in ICD-10
    b. Anankastic personalities are excessively pedantic
    c. Religious factors influence antisocial personality disorder
    d. According to DSM-4, conduct disorder should be present before the age of 15 for antisocial personality disorder
    e. Harria-Parmia is a dimension in Cattell's 16PF

84. 18-year-old Jane suffers from anorexia nervosa. Which one of these statements is true about this condition?
    a. Avoidance of carbohydrate rich foods is a criterion
    b. The HPT axis regresses to the pubertal state
    c. Ultrasound shows small ovaries, but a normal sized uterus
    d. Asymptomatic hyperglycaemia is often found
    e. There is an increase in reverse T3 and decreased T4

85. Which one of these statements about bulimia nervosa is correct?

    a. Leucopenia is common

    b. An ICD-10 criterion is a minimum of 2 binges per week over 3 months

    c. The gender ratio is different to that of anorexia

    d. Suicide attempts are seen in 5%

    e. Hypokalaemia and acidosis is seen

86. Tracy has recently given birth to a little boy and has been feeling low. Which one of these statements about this condition is correct?

    a. Puerperal psychosis starts on the 4th or 5th day post-partum

    b. The onset of puerperal psychosis is abrupt

    c. Carbamazepine as a mood stabiliser is unsafe as she is breast-feeding

    d. Maternity blues are not associated with premenstrual tension

    e. Edinburgh Postnatal Depression Scale is observer rated

87. Which one of these statements about severe head injury is correct?

    a. Contralateral optic atrophy is seen in the frontal lobe syndrome

    b. Posterior temporal lobe lesions produce alexia and agraphia

    c. Hypometamorphosis is seen in the Klüver-Bucy syndrome

    d. Posterior parietal lesions cause cortical sensory loss

    e. An occipital lobe lesion will cause ipsilateral homonymous defects with elementary visual hallucination

88. Which one of these statements about aphasia is true?
    a. Retention of repetition only is diagnostic of conduction aphasia
    b. Dysprosody indicates primary motor aphasia
    c. Anomic aphasia is a late symptom of dementia
    d. Right-handers have a better prognosis after CVA involving language processes
    e. Agnosia can be attributed to aphasic misnaming

89. Which one of these statements about Huntingdon's disease is true?
    a. Dementia is of the cortical type
    b. Late onset presents with psychiatric symptoms
    c. Patients do not have symptoms suggestive of agnosia and apraxia
    d. There is astrocytic proliferation and spiny cell loss
    e. GABA is increased in the basal ganglia

90. Which one of the following is suggestive of pseudoseizure?
    a. Normal EEG
    b. Cyanosis
    c. Incontinence of urine
    d. Complete recall for the period of automatism
    e. Past history of GTCS

91. Which one of these statements about schizophrenia is true?
    a. There is a 1% morbid risk in relatives of normal subjects
    b. The prevalence of schizotypal disorder in first degree relatives of schizophrenics is greater than the prevalence of affective disorder
    c. The prevalence of affective disorder in first degree controls is the same as that in first degree relatives of schizophrenics
    d. P300 abnormalities are not seen in unaffected first degree relatives

e. Reversed planum temporale asymmetry is specific to paranoid schizophrenia

92. Which one of the following is a predictor of poor prognosis in schizophrenia?
    a. Female gender
    b. Late onset
    c. Substance abuse
    d. High IQ
    e. Being married

93. A 32-year-old man presents with a long history of anger and suspicion, but no delusion or hallucination. What is this condition known as?
    a. Paraphrenia
    b. Paranoid personality disorder
    c. Paranoid schizophrenia
    d. Negative schizophrenia
    e. Delusional disorder

94. Which one of the following is not a somatic symptom of depression?
    a. Poor appetite
    b. Weight loss
    c. Increased appetite
    d. Hypochondriasis
    e. Hypersomnia

95. Which one of the following drugs does not cause depression?
    a. Erythromycin
    b. Amphetamine
    c. Reserpine
    d. Barbiturate
    e. L-dopa

96. Which one of the following abnormalities occurs in depression?

   a. Decreased 5-HT-2 receptors

   b. Increased H-imipramine binding in platelets

   c. Increased platelet cAMP turnover with stimulation by clonidine

   d. Postsynaptic muscarinic hyposensitivity

   e. Increased monocytes

97. Which one of the following statements is not true regarding seasonal affective disorder?

   a. Diagnosis requires seasonal presentation in at least two successive winter months

   b. There is a phase shift in the normal circadian rhythm of melatonin

   c. There is a melatonin deficit

   d. Mild hypomania is often experienced in summer

   e. Bright light therapy is a treatment option

98. A 29-year-old RAF private presents with vigilance, scanning, motor tension, autonomic hyperactivity and subjective apprehension. What is this condition known as?

   a. Generalised anxiety disorder

   b. Panic disorder

   c. Post-traumatic stress disorder

   d. Acute stress reaction

   e. Depression

99. According to Marks, the following are all characteristics of phobias, except:

   a. Fear is out of proportion to the demands of the situation

   b. Fear cannot be explained

   c. There is an increased predisposition to the startle reflex

   d. Fear leads to avoidance of the fearful situation

   e. Fear is beyond voluntary control

100. Which one of the following is not a common side-effect of donepezil?

   a. Nausea

   b. Vomiting

   c. Diarrhoea

   d. Abdominal pain

   e. Anorexia

101. Which one of these drugs is a partial agonist of the mu opioid receptor?

   a. Pentazocine

   b. Buprenorphine

   c. Naloxone

   d. Naltrexone

   e. Nalorphine

102. Which one of the following associations is not true?

   a. Cocaine – inhibition of reuptake of dopamine

   b. Amphetamine – release of dopamine

   c. MDMA – acute stage sympathomimetic

   d. LSD – increased serotonergic activity

   e. PDP – blocks NMDA associated calcium channels

103. Which one of these statements about the physiology of erection is correct?

   a. The sympathetic system is concerned with maintaining the flaccid state

   b. Sympathetic activity is mediated through the alpha-2 adrenergic system

   c. Parasympathetic stimulation leads to blood flow of about 15 mL/min

   d. NO stimulates guanylate cyclase to convert cyclic guanosine monophosphate into guanosine triphosphate

   e. Sildenafil is an inhibitor of PDE-4

104. Mr Smith develops toenail dystrophy on a mood stabiliser. Which one is he probably taking?
    a. Lithium
    b. Sodium valproate
    c. Carbamazepine
    d. Lamotrigine
    e. Olanzapine

105. The advantages of doing an assessment in the home environment include all, except:
    a. It is more convenient for the doctor
    b. It is more relaxing for the patient
    c. Living conditions can be seen
    d. Social activities can be assessed
    e. Medications can be examined

106. Which one of the following is not a key role of a mental state examination in the elderly?
    a. Assessing sight and hearing difficulties
    b. Assessing anxiety symptoms
    c. Detecting masked depression
    d. Detecting suicidal ideation
    e. Assessing the cognitive state

107. The information/orientation sub-scale of one of the following assessment tools has 12 questions. Which tool is it?
    a. ACE
    b. MMSE
    c. CAPE
    d. CAMCOG
    e. Clock drawing test

108. The cut-off for depression in one of the following scales is 11. Which scale is it?

 a. Geriatric Depression Rating Scale

 b. Beck's Depression Inventory

 c. Brief Assessment Schedule Depression Cards

 d. Montgomery and Aspberg Depression Rating Scale

 e. Hamilton Rating Scale

109. The shortened version of one of the following scales has 143 items and takes 30 minutes to administer. Which scale is it?

 a. CAMCOG

 b. ACE

 c. CARE

 d. GMS

 e. CAPE

110. The number of cases per unit population per unit time is known as:

 a. Incidence

 b. Prevalence

 c. Standardised mortality

 d. Standardised morbidity

 e. QALY

111. A 69-year-old man, living by himself since the death of his wife 3 months ago, is found to have altered speech, daytime drowsiness, clouded consciousness with global impairment (as tested by AMTS), and is feeling perplexed. What is his condition?

 a. Vascular dementia

 b. Lewy Body dementia

 c. Acute and transient psychotic illness

 d. Paraphrenia

 e. Delirium

112. Mr Spencer, a 79-year-old gentleman, had been diagnosed with glaucoma. While on holiday with his wife he was found to have altered consciousness, impaired memory, altered sleep pattern and visual hallucinations. His delirium is most likely due to:

    a. Hypothyroidism
    b. Medication
    c. Stroke
    d. Epilepsy
    e. Renal failure

113. Which one of these statements about the psychosocial aspects of depression is correct?

    a. According to buffer theory, lack of social support directly predisposes to depression
    b. Divorce is the most significant life event according to Holmes and Rahe
    c. Life events are hypothesised to bring forward the onset of depression by 6 months
    d. Loss of a mother before the age of 11 predisposes to adult depression
    e. According to Winokur, antisocial personality disorder (ASPD) belongs to the depressive spectrum disease

114. The antidepressant with the highest affinity for muscarinic receptors in the human brain is:

    a. Amitriptyline
    b. Clomipramine
    c. Desipramine
    d. Amoxapine
    e. Trazodone

115. The most common type of skin reaction caused by tricyclics is:

    a. Exanthema
    b. Urticaria
    c. Erythema multiforme

d. Exfoliative dermatitis

e. Photosensitivity

116. The SSRI with the shortest half-life is:
    a. Citalopram
    b. Fluoxetine
    c. Fluvoxamine
    d. Paroxetine
    e. Sertraline

117. Inhibition by SSRIs of one of the following CYP enzyme systems leads to increased levels of beta-blockers. Which one is it?
    a. 1A2
    b. 2C
    c. 2D6
    d. 3A3
    e. 3A4

118. There is a very low incidence of drug-induced sexual dysfunction in patients treated with:
    a. Paroxetine
    b. Venlafaxine
    c. Ncfazadone
    d. Amitriptyline
    e. Clomipramine

119. Which of these MAOIs inhibits neuronal reuptake of amines?
    a. Phenelzine
    b. Isocarboxazid
    c. Selegiline
    d. Moclobemide
    e. Tranylcypromine

120. Mrs Simpson has not responded to adequate trials of two antidepressants with different profiles. What stage of treatment-resistant depression is she in?

a. Stage 0

b. 1

c. 2

d. 3

e. 4

121. Which one of the following is not a relative contraindication of ECT?

a. Congestive cardiac failure

b. MI within the last six months

c. Poorly controlled epilepsy

d. Asthma

e. Cervical spondylosis

122. Which one of these factors shortens the duration of a seizure during an ECT?

a. Hyperventilation

b. Hypoxygenation

c. Moderate suprathreshold stimulus

d. Younger age

e. Female gender

123. Which one of these statements about dissociative disorders is correct?

a. Dissociative identity disorder present only according to ICD-10

b. Depersonalization disorder is classified under dissociative disorder in ICD-10

c. Dissociative stupor is classified under dissociative disorder in ICD-10 only

d. A diagnosis of dissociative amnesia can be made in the presence of somatisation disorder

e. For a diagnosis of dissociative personality disorder, at least one of the identities or personality states should take control of a person's behaviour

124. Which one of these statements is correct?

a. The most common psychiatric disorder seen in general practice is somatoform disorder

b. Irritable bowel syndrome occurs in 10% of the general population

c. Fibromyalgia affects men more commonly than women

d. The severity of depression in Cushing's syndrome is related to the plasma cortisol level

e. Following MI, CBT plus antidepressant treatment increases the chance of survival more than either one of them on its own

125. Which one of these statements about ICD-10 classification is correct?

a. Sexual dysfunction is part of F6

b. Disorders of sexual preference and gender identity disorders are parts of F6

c. Frotteurism is a disorder of sexual preference

d. Dyspareunia is a diagnostic category

e. Sexual sadism is a diagnostic category

126. Which one of these statements about ethics is correct?

a. The duty-based approach is concerned with balancing judgements about benefit and harm

b. Justice is doing what is best for patients

c. When giving consent, a patient should agree freely to receive the treatment

d. Explicit consent is required when a patient holds out his arm for checking blood pressure

e. Torts are wrongs for which a person is liable in criminal law

127. Which one of the following is not an impulse and habit disorder?

   a. Intermittent explosive disorder

   b. Pathological gambling

   c. Trichotillomania

   d. Episodic dyscontrol syndrome

   e. Kleptomania

128. Which one of the following disorders and countermeasures is not matched correctly?

   a. Paranoid – candour

   b. Histrionic – kind but distant

   c. Obsessive-compulsive – emotional vividness

   d. Schizotypal – conventionality

   e. Borderline – strict boundaries

129. Which one of the following is not an ICD-10 criterion for anorexia nervosa?

   a. Amenorrhoea

   b. Reduced growth hormone

   c. Reduced cortisol

   d. Increased TSH

   e. Increased T4

130. Which one of the following is not a feature of the blood chemistry in anorexia nervosa?

   a. Urea is low in vomiting and laxative misuse

   b. Bicarbonate > 30 mmol/L in laxative misuse

   c. Amylase increased

   d. Carotene decreased

   e. Aspartate transaminase reduced

131. Which one of the following is not a clinical ground for admission following a diagnosis of anorexia?

   a. Petechial rash and platelet suppression

b. Chronicity > 3 years

c. BMI below 13.5 kg/m^2

d. Co-morbidity with impulsive behaviour

e. Intolerable family situation

132. A favourable prognosis in anorexia nervosa is associated with:

a. Lower minimum weight

b. Lower age of onset

c. Personality difficulties

d. Poor relationship with family

e. Social difficulties

133. Which one of the following 'methods' is not included in the DSM-IV criteria for bulimia nervosa?

a. Laxatives

b. Diuretics

c. Strict diet

d. Appetite suppressants

e. Vigorous exercise

Paper 5

1. Which one of these individuals is not a critic of Piaget?
   a. Baillargeon
   b. Donaldson
   c. Winnicott
   d. Bremner
   e. Hood

2. Piaget's theory of lack of transitive inference was disproved by:
   a. Pears and Bryant
   b. Bremner and Bryant
   c. Moore and Fry
   d. Braine and Shanks
   e. Russell and Mitchell

3. In non-paranoid schizophrenia:
   a. Broadbent's early selection of attention does not apply
   b. There is no difficulty in maintaining filtering unlike patients with paranoid schizophrenia,
   c. Most sensory information is lost at a late stage of processing
   d. There is less distraction during dichotic listening
   e. Inefficient filtering contributes to cognitive symptoms

4. The connectionist model of attention is associated with:
   a. Allport
   b. Wickens
   c. Davies
   d. Parasuraman
   e. Rabbitt

5. Adults, when giving electric shocks, were less aggressive when they heard expressions of pain from a victim than when a victim did not make any response. This is an example of:
   a. Catharsis
   b. Empathy
   c. Sympathy
   d. Appeasement ritual
   e. Sadism

6. The age at which a child develops the ability to see three-dimensional space and to accurately judge distances is:
   a. 2 months
   b. 4 months
   c. 6 months
   d. 8 months
   e. 10 months

7. The ability to read words, but not non-words is called:
   a. Surface dyslexia
   b. Double dissociation
   c. Deep dyslexia
   d. Neglect dyslexia
   e. Phonological dyslexia

8. Inability to recognise a familiar face is:
   a. A feature of Gerstmann's syndrome
   b. Known as prosopagnosia
   c. Due to right posterior parietal lobe pathology

    d. The result of a defect in the primal sketch

    e. All of the above

9. Which one of the following factors is not involved in the development of personal relationships?

    a. Physical attractiveness

    b. Sexual attitudes

    c. Complementary attitudes on central issues

    d. Perceived acceptance

    e. Emotional stability

10. Which one of these statements about love is correct?

    a. Lee developed two 13-item scales for love and liking

    b. There are six dimensions in a scale to measure each type of love

    c. Storge is love from friendship

    d. Agape is non-committal love

    e. Ludus is possessive love

11. Which one of these statements about desirable characteristics is correct?

    a. A British sample chose love, trust and mutual respect as important factors in bringing marital satisfaction

    b. Conscientiousness had a significant correlation with interpersonal attraction

    c. Drug-using adolescent friends were similar in self-esteem

    d. The Dyadic Adjustment Scale measures the degree to which partners disagree on various issues

    e. Liking is a function of a number of similar attitudes weighted in terms of their importance

12. Predictors of compatibility between a wife and husband include all except which one of the following:
    a. Extroversion
    b. Personality factors of wife
    c. Lower neuroticism in both
    d. Interest in art
    e. Greater impulse control of wife

13. Which one of these statements is not true with regard to social exchange?
    a. Greater inequity leads to more distress
    b. More distress results in less effort to reduce inequity
    c. Married couples tend to be similar in terms of physical attractiveness as rated by others
    d. There is little evidence to suggest that women trade their physical attractiveness for educational attainment in men
    e. According to the interdependence theory, a relationship would be more satisfying if the outcome was more positive than anticipated

14. Amy's mother points to a pony and teaches her that its name is pony. The next day, Amy spots a sheep and says, 'Pony.' This is an example of:
    a. Over-extension
    b. Pragmatics
    c. Linguistic universals
    d. Holophrastic speech
    e. Transformational grammar

15. A group of people enjoying themselves in the West End are asked for their opinions about the likelihood of tourists to Zimbabwe being attacked by government-backed militia. Most of them significantly over-estimate the risk. This is due to:
    a. Negative transfer effect
    b. Positive transfer effect
    c. Representativeness bias

d. Availability heuristic

e. Convergent thinking

16. Cue exposure for the treatment of alcohol dependence is based on:

a. Covert sensitisation

b. Extinction

c. Aversion

d. Reciprocal inhibition

e. Modelling

17. Two-year-old Alice knows that she is a girl but one day as her dad drives her around in his car she claims that she will grow to be as handsome as her dad. This phenomenon is known as:

a. Gender stability

b. Basic gender identity

c. Gender consistency

d. Electra complex

e. Androgyny

18. A 56-year-old patient who has been in a medium secure unit for more than 15 years sees himself and other patients as inferior to the RMOs and gradually develops low self-esteem. This is due to:

a. Mortification process

b. Institutional view

c. Role-stripping

d. Batch living

e. Moral career

19. A psychiatric trainee has failed the Membership umpteen times and decides to venture into GP training, as Psychiatry is a rubbish discipline. This defence mechanism is known as:

a. Rationalisation

b. Reaction formation

c. Regression

d. Sublimation

e. Displacement

20. Mr Eriksson has recently started an affair with his secretary and been coming home late from work. This has led to a row with his wife and he accuses her of having an affair with her boss. This defence mechanism is known as:

a. Projective identification

b. Acting out

c. Displacement

d. Projection

e. Introjection

21. *The Sun* publishes a news item saying that a 20-year-old woman in Zimbabwe claims that Prince Harry is in love with her and that they have been having an affair. She has previously made news headlines for stalking Brad Pitt who, according to her, was in love with her. What is the name of her condition?

a. Delusion of grandeur

b. Delusion of erotomania

c. Thought insertion

d. Delusion of infidelity

e. Delusion of nihilism

22. A 69-year-old lady with a recent diagnosis of Alzheimer's disease believes that impostors have replaced her husband and son as they now have Martian ears with bristles in them. What is this condition known as?

a. Autochthonous delusion

b. Delusion of reference

c. Delusion of doubles

d. Simultagnosia

e. Prosopagnosia

23. Mr Archer, who has been imprisoned at Bellmarsh, claims that he could hear his conspirators talking in Fulham. What is this condition known as?

a. Thought broadcast

b. Thought insertion

c. Second person auditory hallucination

d. Extracampine hallucination

e. Somatic passivity

24. Mr Kumar, an obese individual, presents with profound daytime somnolence and cyanosis due to hypoventilation. What is the name of his condition?

a. Kleine-Levin syndrome

b. Kluver-Bucy syndrome

c. Pickwickian syndrome

d. Narcolepsy

e. Catalepsy

25. Mrs Williams complains of hearing her daughter playing tennis just before going to sleep. What is this condition called?

a. Hypnagogic hallucination

b. Hypnopompic hallucination

c. Sleep drunkenness

d. Functional hallucination

e. Extracampine auditory hallucination

26. You have diagnosed Mr Roberts with narcolepsy. Which of the following is not likely to be a feature of his condition?
    a. Episodes of irresistible sleep during the day
    b. Falling down when told his mother has cancer
    c. Episodes of sleep lasting for 30 minutes
    d. Normal CT brain
    e. Hypnopompic hallucinations

27. Which one of these statements about night terror is correct ?
    a. There is relative amnesia on waking
    b. It occurs in REM sleep
    c. It occurs in persons suffering from somnambulism
    d. It occurs when the person is about to wake up
    e. It can be used in the law as insane automatism

28. When under hypnosis, John would do all the following, except:
    a. Cease to make his plans
    b. Reject his distortions
    c. Have increased suggestibility
    d. Readily enact unusual roles
    e. Remember repressed but not suppressed memories

29. A 19-year-old boy is anxious despite having expelled (from his conscious perception) thoughts of killing his brother. This process is known as:
    a. Repression
    b. Suppression
    c. Regression
    d. Isolation
    e. Denial

30. All the following associations are true, except:
    a. Winnicott – libidinal object
    b. Fairburn – ideal object
    c. Klein – paranoid-schizoid position

    d. Adler – masculine protest

    e. Meyer – psychobiology

31. Which of the following activities is not goal directed?

    a. Stereotypy

    b. Tics

    c. Mannerisms

    d. Chorea

    e. Hemiballismus

32. A form of perseveration is:

    a. Logorrhoea

    b. Logoclonia

    c. Witzelsucht

    d. Verbigeration

    e. Verstimmung

33. Which of the following is not a formal thought disorder type described by Schneider?

    a. Derailment

    b. Drivelling

    c. Concrete thinking

    d. Omission

    e. Fusion

34. Which one of these statements about behavioural treatments is correct?

    a. Habituation is the use of exposure without response prevention

    b. Reciprocal inhibition means that as relaxation inhibits anxiety they are mutually inclusive

    c. In shaping, successively closer approximations to the desired behaviour are reinforced

    d. In chaining, the components of a more simple behaviour are first taught and connected to obtain the desired behaviour

    e. None of the above

35. Which one of the following is not included in Gestalt psychology?
   a. Law of simplicity
   b. Law of continuity
   c. Law of primacy
   d. Figure ground differentiation
   e. Law of proximity

36. Which of these statements about the visual cliff experiment is correct?
   a. It demonstrates height perception in an infant
   b. It demonstrates depth perception in an infant
   c. It can be used with an infant from 6 weeks of age
   d. It implies a two-dimensional percept from a two-dimensional retinal image
   e. It differentiates organic and functional disorders

37. Which of these statements about explicit memory is not true?
   a. It involves the entorhinal cortex
   b. It includes declarative memory
   c. Memory passes from the cortex to the medial temporal lobe for storage
   d. Declarative and episodic memory are probably stored independently
   e. It is a type of long-term memory

38. Which of these statements about implicit memory is correct?
   a. It can be learned fast
   b. It requires the cerebellum
   c. It is factual memory
   d. Only classical learning is involved
   e. Only operant learning is involved

39. The auditory association cortex is located in the:
   a. Dorso-lateral frontal lobe on the dominant side

b. Medial temporal lobe

c. Inferior parietal lobe

d. Medial frontal cortices

e. Dorso-lateral frontal lobes bilaterally

40. In aphasia caused by damage to Wernicke's area:

a. Dysphonia is a feature

b. Speech has abnormal prosody

c. Speech has abnormal tone

d. Written words cannot be understood

e. Broca's area is spared

41. Which of the following is not a consequence of damage to the arcuate fasciculus?

a. Comprehension is intact

b. Verbal fluency is intact

c. Repetition is impaired

d. Repetition is preserved

e. Kluver-Bucy syndrome

42. Pseudoagnosia is caused by a lesion at which one of the following locations?

a. Occipital lobe

b. Inferior temporal lobe

c. Dominant parietal lobe

d. Non-dominant parietal lobe

e. Bilateral parietal lobe

43. Balint's syndrome involves:

a. Apperceptive agnosia

b. Simultagnosia

c. Prosopagnosia

d. Autotopagnosia

e. Semantic agnosia

44. Visual agnosia is caused by damage to the:
   a. Left occipital lobe
   b. Right occipital lobe
   c. Left parietal lobe
   d. Right parietal lobe
   e. Left frontal association cortex

45. Which one of these statements about Gerstmann's syndrome is not true?
   a. There is a form of developmental Gerstmann's syndrome in children
   b. In adults, it may present with aphasia
   c. In adults, many symptoms fade with time
   d. It is caused by damage to the infra-marginal gyri
   e. It causes left-right disorientation

46. Which one of these statements about apraxia is not true?
   a. Lipermann introduced the concept 'apraxia of speech'
   b. Limb-kinetic apraxia results from the loss of hand-finger dexterity
   c. Ideomotor apraxia is caused by damage to the left hemisphere
   d. Constructional apraxia is caused by damage to the left cerebral hemisphere
   e. Apraxia of eyelid opening is caused by inhibited levator palpebrae

47. Which of the following associations is not true?
   a. Positive and negative symptoms – Reynolds
   b. Concrete thinking – Goldstein
   c. Over-inclusive thinking – Cameron
   d. Range of convenience – Kelly
   e. Alogia – Kraeplin

48. 'The salt cellar was pushed toward the Irishman but before it could reach him he knew he must return to his home to greet the Pope, as our Lord was going to be born again to one of the women.' What is this type of thinking known as?

a. Delusional intuition

b. Delusional perception

c. Functional delusion

d. Synaesthesia

e. Reflex hallucination

49. A 24-year-old man reported the following experience. He heard voices saying 'GT is a bloody paradox'; 'He is that, he should be locked up'; and 'He is not, he is a lovely man.' This phenomenon is known as:

a. Echo de la pensee

b. Gedankenlautwerden

c. Second person auditory hallucination

d. Running commentary

e. Third person auditory hallucination

50. 'I feel my hand going up to salute, and my lips mouthing Heil Hitler . . . I have to try very hard to stop my arm from going up.' This phenomenon is known as:

a. Somatic passivity

b. Passivity of impulse

c. Passivity of volition

d. Passivity of affect

e. Thought insertion

51. 'Rays from the sun are directed by army satellites in an intense beam, which I can feel entering the centre of my knee and then radiating outwards causing pain.' This phenomenon is known as:

a. Somatic passivity

b. Passivity of impulse

c. Passivity of volition

d. Passivity of affect

e. Thought insertion

52. According to Brown and Harris, the following are all risk factors for depression, except:

a. Lack of close confidant

b. Loss of mother before the age of 11

c. Living in an inner-city area

d. Three or more children under the age of 14 at home

e. No employment outside the home

53. According to Hamilton, the third most common symptom of depression in males is:

a. Loss of interest

b. Psychic anxiety

c. Initial insomnia

d. Suicide

e. Guilt

54. Mr Greenwich presents with hilarity, loss of thoughts and motor retardation. The most likely diagnosis is:

a. Reactive depression

b. Endogenous depression

c. Mania

d. Agitated depression

e. Manic stupor

55. Mrs Martin presents with a relapse of bipolar affective disorder. Mental state assessment reveals an incessant need to talk and express her thoughts. This phenomenon is known as:

a. Loosening of association

b. Flight of ideas

c. Drivelling

d. Pressure of speech

e. Verbigeration

56. Which of the following associations is not true?

a. Schizophreniform states – Langfeldt

b. Schizoaffective psychosis – Kasanin

c. Benign stupor – Hoch

d. Recovered schizophrenics – Kraepelin

e. Schizophrenia – Bleuler

57. Which of the following associations is not true?

a. Self psychology – mirror transference

b. Supportive psychotherapy – therapist actively offers advice

c. Brief psychodynamic psychotherapy – focalisation of the conflict

d. Analytic psychotherapy – collective unconscious

e. Transactional analysis – positive regard

58. The defence mechanism linked with dissociative disorders is:

a. Undoing

b. Displacement

c. Suppression

d. Regression

e. Identification

59. Negative automatic thoughts include all, except:
   a. Selective abstraction
   b. Arbitrary inference
   c. Over-generalisation
   d. Minimisation
   e. Catastrophisation

60. Pseudohallucinations are seen in:
   a. Personality disorder
   b. Postpartum psychosis
   c. Bipolar affective disorder
   d. Bereavement
   e. Normal sleep

61. Which of the following terms is not associated with Jung?
   a. Collective unconscious
   b. Archetype
   c. Old man
   d. Animus
   e. Inferiority complex

62. A 29-year-old lady with a first episode of depression was started on an antidepressant by her GP and subsequently referred to you as she had developed a headache and reduced appetite. Which antidepressant had she most likely been given?
   a. Paroxetine
   b. Sertraline
   c. Fluoxetine
   d. Citalopram
   e. Escitalopram

63. A 72-year-old man develops UTI since being on an antidepressant. He also suffers from prostatism. Which antidepressant is most likely responsible?

   a. Trazodone

   b. Nefazadone

   c. Mirtazapine

   d. Amitriptyline

   e. Reboxetine

64. A 28-year-old lady develops an episode of depression following an emergency Caesarean section. She has started breast-feeding her baby, so a suitable antidepressant for her would be:

   a. Citalopram

   b. Sertraline

   c. Fluoxetine

   d. Amitriptyline

   e. Mirtazapine

65. A 24-year-old woman in the first trimester of pregnancy develops a severe depressive episode with biological symptoms and suicidal thoughts. Which is the safest antidepressant to prescribe?

   a. Fluoxetine

   b. Paroxetine

   c. Sertraline

   d. Citalopram

   e. Escitalopram

66. A 36-year-old man with a long history of recurrent depressive disorders has become dependent on his antidepressant medication. Which is it most likely to be?

   a. Moclobemide

   b. Phenelzine

   c. Tranylcypromine

   d. Fluvoxamine

   e. Escitalopram

67. Diazepam:

a. Has an inactive metabolite called desmethyldiazepam

b. Has 95% protein binding

c. Absorption is increased by the presence of food

d. Half-life is 12 hours

e. Does not cause blurred vision

68. Which one of these statements about benzodiazepines is correct?

a. Lorazepam has less receptor affinity than diazepam

b. Lorazepam is more lipid soluble than diazepam

c. Oral diazepam has 50% bioavailability

d. The active metabolite of flurazepam has a half-life of 120 hours

e. Lorazepam has less receptor affinity than oxazepam

69. Flumazenil:

a. Is an inverse agonist at GABA receptors

b. Is an epileptogenic drug

c. Is a partial agonist at GABA receptors

d. Reduces panic and is therefore a pharmacological test for panic disorder

e. Has an elimination half-life of 4 hours

70. Which one of these statements about benzodiazepines is correct?

a. They suppress stage 2 and 3 sleep

b. Withdrawal causes hyperacusis

c. Tolerance to their anxiolytic effect is greater than to their amnestic effect

d. Tolerance is least to anticonvulsant properties

e. 8% of patients have hallucination on withdrawal from benzodiazepine

71. Buspirone:
    a. Causes muscle relaxation
    b. Is an antagonist at 5-HT-1A sites
    c. Is a postsynaptic dopamine antagonist
    d. Is a cause of reduced seizure threshold
    e. Is an azaspirodecanedione

72. Flupenthixol is a type of:
    a. Aliphatic phenothiazine
    b. Piperazine phenothiazine
    c. Piperidine phenothiazine
    d. Thioxanthene
    e. Diphenylbutylpiperidine

73. Which one of the following is not a parenteral route of administration?
    a. Intramuscular
    b. Rectal
    c. Subcutaneous
    d. Topical
    e. Inhalational

74. Which one of the following factors enhances the absorption of IM haloperidol?
    a. Lipid solubility
    b. Low molecular mass
    c. Physical exercise
    d. Cardiac failure
    e. Emotional excitement

75. A high percentage of amitriptyline is present in the unbound form in:

a. Renal disease

b. Carcinoma

c. Hypothyroidism

d. Burns

e. Malnutrition

76. The most common type of reaction involved in hepatic phase 1 biotransformation is:

a. Reduction

b. Conjugation

c. Hydrolysis

d. Oxidation

e. Demethylation

77. Mr Davies presented with a rapidly progressive dementia and abnormal movements. On EEG, you find triphasic waves. The most likely diagnosis is:

a. Dementia in Huntingdon's disease

b. Dementia in Parkinson's disease

c. Dementia in Lewy body disease

d. Dementia in Creutzfeldt-Jacob disease (CJD)

e. Dementia in HIV

78. Mrs Chandler has experienced brief episodes of psychotic and depressive illness in the past and there is a history of dementia in her grandfather and father. She is starting to show cognitive impairment, but much earlier than when the disease started in her father. The probable diagnosis is:

a. Dementia in Lewy body disease

b. Alzheimer's disease

c. Binswanger's disease

d. Shy-Drager syndrome

e. Dementia in Huntingdon's disease

79. Mr Henry, a 20-year-old Afro-Caribbean male is assessed under Section 2 of MHA. He presents with a silly smile and continues to stare at himself in a mirror whilst you talk to him. His speech is incoherent. What is the name of his condition?

   a. Paranoid schizophrenia
   b. Residual schizophrenia
   c. Catatonia
   d. Hebephrenia
   e. Schizoaffective disorder

80. Brain autopsy of a middle-aged man with dementia showed loss of GABAergic neurons in the striatum and atrophy of the caudate nucleus and putamen along with increased dopaminergic pigmentation in the basal ganglia. The diagnosis is:

   a. Dementia in Lewy body disease
   b. Dementia in Parkinson's disease
   c. Dementia in Huntingdon's disease
   d. Progressive supranuclear palsy
   e. Pick's disease

81. Mrs Darling, a 32-year-old housewife, presents with repeated episodes of acute anxiety and is very concerned about travelling away from home by herself, especially on trains and buses. The diagnosis is:

   a. Generalised anxiety disorder
   b. Panic disorder
   c. Specific phobia
   d. Social phobia
   e. Anxiety disorder NOS

82. Mr Fergusson, a 69-year-old man, presents with delirium following surgery for a spinal injury. In this condition, which one of the following statements is true?

    a. Nominal dysphasia is uncommon

    b. The level of alertness is abnormally low or high

    c. A normal CSF rules out CJD

    d. A PTA between 1 and 24 hours is severe

    e. There will be no disturbance in his sleep-wake cycle

83. Which one of the following is true of congenital disorders?

    a. Friedreich's ataxia has autosomal recessive inheritance

    b. Dystrophia myotonica has X-linked inheritance

    c. Duchenne muscular dystrophy has X-linked dominant inheritance

    d. Wilson's disease has autosomal dominant inheritance

    e. Narcolepsy is associated with autosomal dominant inheritance and HLA-DR4 antigen

84. Mr Rodin suffers from Gilles de la Tourette syndrome. Which of the following statements about this condition is true?

    a. Mean age of onset is 11 years

    b. It is less commonly associated with obsessionality

    c. Association with ADD is 10%

    d. Self-injurious behaviour occurs in 5%

    e. SPECT shows hyperperfusion in the frontal cortex and hypoperfusion in the temporal cortex

85. Mr Franklin has a long history of alcohol dependence. Which one of the following statements about this condition is true?

    a. Withdrawal hallucinations occur after 48 hours of abstinence

    b. Second person auditory hallucinations are common during withdrawal

    c. Convergent gaze palsy is seen in Wernicke's disease

    d. Primary memory is lost in Korsakoff's syndrome

    e. REM sleep increases after alcohol intoxication

86. Mrs Balham has been diagnosed with Alzheimer's disease and her son is interested in knowing the prognostic factors. Which one of the following features is associated with poor survival?
    a. Parietal lobe damage
    b. Female gender
    c. Late age of onset
    d. Lack of wandering
    e. Absence of apraxia

87. Which one of these statements is not true with regard to Alzheimer's disease?
    a. Depression occurs up to 50% in patients
    b. EEG shows slowing of alpha and beta waves
    c. Chromosome 14 is implicated in approximately 75% of cases of early onset familial Alzheimer's disease
    d. There is an increase in muscarinic M2 receptors
    e. Neuropathological diagnosis requires more than 10 plaques in people between ages of 66 and 75 years

88. Neurofibrillary tangles occur in all, except:
    a. Progressive supranuclear palsy
    b. CJD
    c. Pick's disease
    d. Lewy body disease
    e. Dementia pugilistica

89. Neuroimaging reveals deep white matter lesions in all the following conditions, except:
    a. Depression
    b. CJD
    c. Multiple sclerosis
    d. Hydrocephalus
    e. Binswanger's disease

90. Which one of the following histological changes is not seen in the brain of patients suffering from Pick's disease?
    a. Neurofibrillary tangles
    b. Hirano bodies
    c. Amyloid deposition
    d. All of the above
    e. None of the above

91. Mrs Milner is a 70-year-old lady presenting with late paraphrenia. Which of these statements about this condition is correct?
    a. Depression is associated with hyperactivity and dysregulation of HPA axis
    b. Persecutory delusions are found in 50% of patients
    c. First rank symptoms are rarely seen
    d. Grandiosity delusions are rare
    e. Degenerative hearing impairment is a risk factor

92. Which of the following is not a physiological effect of reduced pCO_2 ?
    a. Bradycardia
    b. Reduced availability of oxygen in oxyhaemoglobin
    c. Vasoconstriction of cerebral arteries
    d. Increased irritability of autonomic sensory and motor systems
    e. Bronchoconstriction

93. Which one of the following factors is not thought to be a cause of PTSD?
    a. Lower basal cortisol levels
    b. Increased catecholamines
    c. Small hippocampus
    d. Decreased HPA activity
    e. Prior history of psychiatric illness

94. Rat man is associated with:

a. Hysteria

b. OCD

c. Schizophrenia

d. Melancholia

e. Manic depressive psychosis

95. A 32-year-old man presents with a long history of attention seeking, lack of empathy and being exploitative. What type of personality disorder does he have?

a. Histrionic

b. Paranoid

c. Narcissistic

d. Dissocial

e. Emotionally unstable

96. Which of these combinations of subunits make up the GABA-BZ receptor complex?

a. 2 alpha-1, 2 beta-2 and 1 gamma-1

b. 2 alpha-2, 2 beta-2 and 2 gamma-2

c. 2 alpha-1, 1 beta-2 and 1 gamma-1

d. 2 alpha-1, 2 beta-2 and 1 gamma-2

e. 2 alpha-1, 2 beta-2 and 1 gamma-2

97. Which one of these statements about benzodiazepine drug use and pregnancy is correct?

a. Cleft-lip and cleft-palate is associated with maternal benzodiazepine use

b. Benzodiazepine taken late in pregnancy does not cause feeding difficulties in the baby

c. Benzodiazepine taken late in pregnancy does not cause respiratory depression in the baby

d. In an infant, benzodiazepine withdrawal does not start 2 weeks after its birth

e. Developmental dysmorphism similar to foetal alcohol syndrome has not been described

98. Which one of these statements about benzodiazepines and tolerance is correct?

    a. Tolerance readily develops to the anxiolytic properties of benzodiazepines, thereby limiting their use in GAD

    b. There is cross tolerance between benzodiazepines, but no cross tolerance between benzodiazepines and barbiturates

    c. A clockwise hysteresis curve is obtained when the effects of benzodiazepines are plotted against time

    d. Tolerance to all effects of benzodiazepines ends within 8–10 weeks

    e. Tolerance to sedative effects is pronounced within 1 week

99. Which one of these statements about benzodiazepines is correct?

    a. When discontinuing benzodiazepines, dosage should be reduced over 1–4 months

    b. Phobic symptoms predict a good response to treatment with benzodiazepines

    c. Guidelines recommend continuous use for a short period of 2–4 weeks

    d. In the UK, 40% of benzodiazepines are prescribed to women

    e. Neurological problems from long-term use of benzodiazepines resolve completely

100. Mrs Jones had a seizure episode after being started on one of the following medications for management of anxiety disorder. Which one is it likely to be?

    a. Propranolol

    b. Zolpidem

    c. Zaleplon

    d. Buspirone

    e. Paroxetine

101. Which one of the following drugs is a tertiary amine?

    a. Imipramine

    b. Desipramine

c. Nortriptyline

d. Dothiepin

e. Lofepramine

102. All but one of the following drugs are commonly associated with delirium. Which is the exception?

a. Salbutamol inhaler

b. Digoxin

c. Diuretics

d. NSAIDs

e. Selegiline

103. Which of the following scales has items pertaining to the aetiology and course?

a. Delirium Symptom Interview

b. Confusement Assessment Method questionnaire

c. Delirium Rating Scale

d. Confusional State Evaluation

e. Informant Questionnaire on the Cognitive Decline in the Elderly

104. A 50-year-old man presents with mood change, personality changes and normal EEG. The most likely diagnosis is:

a. CJD

b. Lewy body disease

c. Dementia pugilistica

d. Pick's disease

e. Whipple's disease

105. The frontal lobe type of dementia is associated with:

a. Whipple's disease

b. Dementia pugilistica

c. Normal pressure hydrocephalus

d. Progressive supranuclear palsy

e. Motor neurone disease

106. NINCDS-ADRDA criteria for probable Alzheimer's disease include all, except:

a. Atypical features in the presence of systemic disease

b. Age between 40 and 90

c. Associated psychiatric symptoms

d. Family history of dementia

e. Normal CT scan

107. Regarding genetics of Alzheimer's disease, the following statement/s could be true: Presenilin gene is located on

a. Chromosome 14

b. Chromosome 1

c. Chromosome 21

d. Chromosome 19

e. Chromosome 2

108. Hirano bodies are seen in all, except:

a. Alzheimer's disease

b. Parkinson's disease

c. Pick's disease

d. Amyotrophic lateral sclerosis

e. Ageing

109. Granulo-vacuolar degeneration is seen in all, except:

a. Ageing

b. Alzheimer's disease

c. Down syndrome

d. Lewy body disease

e. Progressive supranuclear palsy

110. A histological globoid-eosinophilic structure surrounded by blue halo is:

a. Amyloid protein

b. Granulo-vacuolar degeneration

c. Hirano body

d. Lewy body

e. Astrocytes

111. Which one of these neurotransmitters is probably not present in cortical neurones?

a. Acetylcholine

b. GABA

c. Glutamate

d. Somatostatin

e. CRF

112. A 69-year-old man with no history of hypertension presents with abrupt onset of focal neurological signs and uneven impairment of cognitive dysfunction. What is the name of his condition?

a. Vascular dementia

b. Multi-infarct dementia

c. Sub-cortical vascular dementia

d. Alzheimer's disease

e. Binswanger's disease

113. The following are scored 2 on the Hachinski ischaemia score, except:

a. Focal neurological symptoms

b. Focal neurological signs

c. Atherosclerosis

d. History of hypertension

e. Fluctuating course

114. A 43-year-old gentleman presents with a history of migraine, recurrent stroke, pseudobulbar palsy and subcortical dementia. What is the name of his condition?

a. Binswanger's disease

b. Progressive supranuclear palsy

c. Amyotrophic lateral sclerosis

d. CADASIL

e. Huntington's disease

115. Factors that reduce seizure threshold during ECT include all, except:

    a. Sensory stimulation

    b. Reserpine

    c. Lignocaine

    d. Female gender

    e. Young age

116. Which one of these statements about stereotactic subcaudate tractotomy is correct?

    a. It involves interruption of the anterior limb of the internal capsule bilaterally

    b. It involves interruption of association fibres from the orbital frontal cortex

    c. It requires a sequence of treatments

    d. The target site is the lower medial quadrant of the frontal lobe

    e. Haemorrhage is uncommon, but 1–2% develop personality changes

117. 'My boss laughed at two typing errors I had made in a draft because he thinks I am a poor typist.' The concept applied is:

    a. Selective abstraction

    b. Arbitrary inference

    c. Overgeneralisation

    d. Magnification

    e. Personalisation

118. Which of the following is a preventative strategy used in CBT for depression?

    a. Activity scheduling

    b. Challenging negative automatic thoughts

    c. Challenging assumptions

    d. Graded task assignment

    e. Identifying negative automatic thoughts

119. 'Demence precoce' was coined by:
   a. Griesinger
   b. Haslam
   c. Morel
   d. Kraepelin
   e. Kahlbaum

120. 'A sort of an intercourse as if a man was really there. He was not there of course . . . but it was as if a man was with me . . . that is what I felt.' This phenomenon is:
   a. Made will
   b. Made affect
   c. Made impulse
   d. Somatic passivity
   e. Somatic hallucination

121. The following are manifestations of thought disorder due to an unstable goal, except:
   a. Tangentiality
   b. Derailment
   c. Distractibility
   d. Perseveration
   e. Blocking

122. According to Crow, Type 2 schizophrenia is characterised by which one of the following features:
   a. Acute onset
   b. Positive symptoms
   c. Formal thought disorder
   d. Biochemical imbalance
   e. Structural abnormalities of brain

123. Factors indicating poor prognosis in schizophrenia include all, except:

a. Poor pre-morbid adjustment

b. Family history of affective disorder

c. Insidious onset

d. Onset in adolescence

e. Enlargement of cerebral ventricles

124. Largactil is a drug of which class:

a. Aliphatic phenothiazine

b. Piperidine phenothiazine

c. Piperazine phenothiazine

d. Diphenylbutylpiperidine

e. Thioxanthene

125. Which one of these statements about bulimia nervosa is correct?

a. BITE is observer rated

b. Shoplifting is more common than promiscuity

c. 50% of female alcoholics have a history of eating disorder

d. CBT is gold standard when given individually but not as a group

e. Mixed anorexia and bulimia is associated with a better outcome

126. James experiences sensory aura with tingling, numbness, visual distortions and formed hallucinations. These symptoms suggest a lesion in the:

a. Temporal lobe

b. Frontal lobe

c. Parietal lobe

d. Occipital lobe

e. Brain stem

127. Mr Mason has a history of epilepsy and hamartoma and presents with psychosis 15 years following the onset of epilepsy. The diagnosis is:

a. Ictal psychosis

b. Post-ictal psychosis

c. Chronic inter-ictal psychosis

d. Pre-ictal psychosis

e. Psychosis unrelated to epilepsy

128. Which one of the following features is not often found in non-epileptic seizures?

a. Family history of psychiatric disorder

b. Stereotyped attack pattern

c. Left-sided somato-sensory symptoms

d. Affective disorder

e. Deliberate self-harm

129. Perry presents with headache, poor concentration, fluctuating memory loss, unequal pupils and normal optic discs. The diagnosis is:

a. Subarachnoid haemorrhage

b. Subdural haematoma

c. Migraine

d. Dementia

e. Motor neurone disease

130. Ken presents with delayed relaxation of skeletal muscles, slowly progressive weakness and wasting, cataract, hypogonadism and frontal balding. The diagnosis is:

a. Friedrich's ataxia

b. Duchenne muscular dystrophy

c. Dystrophia myotonica

d. Myasthenia gravis

e. Motor neurone disease

131. Sven presents with rapid cognitive deterioration, delusional psychosis, catatonia and stupor. The diagnosis is:
    a. Frontal lobe tumour
    b. Temporal lobe tumour
    c. Parietal lobe tumour
    d. Occipital lobe tumour
    e. Corpus callosum tumour

132. Which of these metals causes toxic effects that resemble CJD?
    a. Aluminium
    b. Arsenic
    c. Bismuth
    d. Gold
    e. Lead

133. Psychosis accompanied by hair loss, parotid enlargement, skin lesions and Mees lines is consistent with poisoning by which of the following metals?
    a. Mercury
    b. Nickel
    c. Thallium
    d. Tin
    e. Zinc

134. John presents with erethism, characterised by the inability to function in front of observers, timidity, and nervousness with strangers. These symptoms are consistent with poisoning by:
    a. Lead
    b. Manganese
    c. Arsenic
    d. Mercury
    e. Vanadium

135. Which one of these statements about thyroid function is correct?

a. Normal TSH excludes hypothyroidism due to hypothalamic disease

b. EEG shows slowing of the dominant rhythm and increased background activity in hypothyroidism

c. When lithium is stopped, its effects on thyroid function reverse in 1–2 months

d. Younger patients present with apathetic hyperthyroidism

e. T3 toxicosis is a late phenomenon

136. HRNB includes all, except:

a. MMPI

b. WAIS-R

c. Trail Making Test

d. Stroop Colour–Word Interference Test

e. Category Test

Answers

Paper 1

1. c	2. b	3. b	4. b	5. c	6. b	7. c	8. a
9. c	10. c	11. b	12. b	13. c	14. a	15. c	16. b
17. c	18. d	19. b	20. b	21. b	22. c	23. a	24. e
25. a	26. b	27. c	28. d	29. c	30. b	31. c	32. b
33. d	34. e	35. a	36. c	37. d	38. e	39. a	40. b
41. a	42. e	43. c	44. c	45. e	46. a	47. d	48. a
49. b	50. d	51. e	52. a	53. d	54. a	55. b	56. d
57. b	58. b	59. b	60. b	61. d	62. d	63. b	64. d
65. a	66. c	67. d	68. c	69. d	70. b	71. b	72. b
73. c	74. a	75. e	76. a	77. b	78. a	79. b	80. d
81. e	82. c	83. b	84. c	85. e	86. b	87. d	88. c
89. c	90. b	91. a	92. c	93. d	94. e	95. a	96. a
97. d	98. a	99. b	100. b	101. e	102. a	103. d	104. a
105. c	106. a	107. e	108. e	109. a	110. c	111. d	112. b
113. b	114. d	115. d	116. c	117. b	118. b	119. b	120. c
121. c	122. b	123. d	124. e	125. a	126. a	127. c	128. b
129. c	130. c	131. d	132. c	133. c	134. a	135. d	136. b

Paper 2

1. d	2. a	3. b	4. d	5. e	6. d	7. c	8. e
9. c	10. d	11. a	12. a	13. c	14. b	15. b	16. b
17. c	18. d	19. e	20. a	21. d	22. c	23. a	24. a
25. a	26. d	27. c	28. c	29. c	30. e	31. d	32. d
33. d	34. b	35. a	36. b	37. b	38. b	39. d	40. c
41. c	42. b	43. e	44. c	45. e	46. d	47. e	48. d
49. a	50. d	51. c	52. d	53. b	54. b	55. a	56. b
57. d	58. d	59. e	60. d	61. b	62. b	63. c	64. b
65. c	66. d	67. d	68. d	69. c	70. e	71. b	72. d
73. b	74. a	75. e	76. d	77. e	78. d	79. a	80. d
81. a	82. b	83. e	84. c	85. a	86. d	87. a	88. c
89. a	90. e	91. e	92. e	93. d	94. c	95. e	96. e
97. d	98. d	99. a	100. d	101. c	102. c	103. a	104. c
105. c	106. d	107. a	108. d	109. c	110. b	111. e	112. b
113. e	114. a	115. c	116. d	117. e	118. d	119. c	120. c
121. b	122. e	123. d	124. d	125. b	126. c	127. c	128. a
129. d	130. c	131. a	132. a	133. b	134. b	135. a	

Paper 3

1. e	2. d	3. a	4. d	5. b	6. b	7. b	8. e
9. c	10. a	11. b	12. c	13. b	14. c	15. b	16. c
17. d	18. d	19. a	20. c	21. d	22. e	23. a	24. b
25. d	26. e	27. b	28. b	29. b	30. c	31. c	32. c
33. a	34. a	35. a	36. b	37. d	38. b	39. b	40. d
41. a	42. e	43. d	44. e	45. d	46. d	47. c	48. e
49. a	50. d	51. b	52. c	53. b	54. d	55. a	56. c
57. d	58. b	59. c	60. a	61. c	62. e	63. a	64. d
65. b	66. d	67. c	68. b	69. d	70. c	71. a	72. e
73. d	74. d	75. b	76. c	77. b	78. c	79. a	80. c
81. d	82. b	83. b	84. c	85. c	86. c	87. a	88. c
89. d	90. a	91. d	92. a	93. e	94. e	95. b	96. e
97. d	98. e	99. d	100. c	101. c	102. b	103. d	104. b
105. c	106. e	107. d	108. a	109. e	110. c	111. c	112. c
113. b	114. d	115. e	116. b	117. d	118. b	119. a	120. e
121. b	122. b	123. b	124. a	125. c	126. b	127. a	128. c
129. e	130. e	131. c	132. c	133. d	134. b	135. b	

Paper 4

1. e	2. e	3. b	4. c	5. d	6. a	7. a	8. d
9. e	10. d	11. d	12. d	13. c	14. e	15. b	16. e
17. b	18. c	19. c	20. b	21. b	22. d	23. c	24. d
25. c	26. b	27. c	28. b	29. b	30. d	31. b	32. c
33. d	34. b	35. c	36. c	37. e	38. c	39. c	40. a
41. a	42. a	43. b	44. d	45. b	46. d	47. b	48. a
49. a	50. b	51. c	52. d	53. c	54. c	55. e	56. c
57. d	58. d	59. c	60. c	61. c	62. c	63. d	64. a
65. d	66. e	67. c	68. c	69. e	70. d	71. a	72. d
73. c	74. c	75. b	76. e	77. a	78. b	79. c	80. b
81. e	82. d	83. a	84. e	85. e	86. a	87. b	88. b
89. c	90. c	91. c	92. c	93. b	94. d	95. a	96. e
97. a	98. a	99. c	100. d	101. b	102. d	103. a	104. a
105. a	106. a	107. c	108. a	109. c	110. a	111. e	112. b
113. e	114. a	115. a	116. d	117. c	118. c	119. e	120. c
121. b	122. b	123. c	124. b	125. b	126. c	127. d	128. b
129. a	130. c	131. b	132. b	133. d			

Paper 5

1. c	2. a	3. e	4. a	5. b	6. c	7. e	8. b
9. c	10. c	11. b	12. e	13. b	14. a	15. d	16. b
17. b	18. e	19. a	20. d	21. b	22. c	23. d	24. c
25. a	26. e	27. c	28. b	29. d	30. a	31. c	32. b
33. c	34. c	35. c	36. a	37. c	38. b	39. b	40. d
41. c	42. a	43. b	44. a	45. d	46. d	47. e	48. b
49. e	50. b	51. a	52. c	53. b	54. e	55. d	56. d
57. e	58. e	59. d	60. d	61. e	62. c	63. d	64. b
65. a	66. c	67. b	68. d	69. b	70. b	71. e	72. d
73. b	74. d	75. c	76. d	77. d	78. e	79. d	80. c
81. b	82. b	83. a	84. a	85. c	86. a	87. d	88. b
89. b	90. d	91. a	92. a	93. d	94. b	95. c	96. d
97. a	98. c	99. a	100. d	101. a	102. a	103. c	104. d
105. e	106. a	107. a	108. b	109. c	110. d	111. a	112. a
113. d	114. d	115. c	116. d	117. b	118. c	119. c	120. e
121. e	122. e	123. b	124. a	125. b	126. c	127. c	128. b
129. a	130. c	131. e	132. c	133. c	134. d	135. c	136. d

References

Johnstone E, Lawrie S, Cunningham-Owens D *et al. Companion to Psychiatric Studies*. 7th ed. Edinburgh: Churchill Livingstone; 2004.

Puri B, Hall A. *Revision Notes in Psychiatry*. 2nd ed. London: Hodder Arnold; 2004.

Tantam D, Birchwood M, editors. *Seminars in Psychology and the Social Sciences*. London: Gaskell (Royal College of Psychiatrists); 1994.

King D, editor. *Seminars in Clinical Psychopharmacology*. 2nd ed. London: Gaskell (Royal College of Psychiatrists); 2004.

Butler R, Pitt B, editors. *Seminars in Old Age Psychiatry*. London: Gaskell (Royal College of Psychiatrists); 1998.

Stein G, Wilkinson G, editors. *Seminars in General Adult Psychiatry*. 2nd ed. London: Gaskell (Royal College of Psychiatrists); 2007.

Gelder M, Cowen P, Harrison P. *Shorter Oxford Textbook of Psychiatry*. 5th ed. Oxford: Oxford University Press; 2006.

Sims A. *Symptoms in the Mind*. Revised ed. Philadelphia: WB Saunders Co Ltd; 2002.

Index

Key: (Q) = question; (A) = answer